TESTIMONIA

RE: Permanent Diabetes Control (bool

Dr. Konduru is an intelligent and committed scientist who has learned to manage his diabetes and cardiovascular risk factors. This book represents a comprehensive and readable review that could help many people with diabetes.

Dr. Marshall Dahl
BSc, MD, PhD, FRCPC, Certified Endocrinologist
Faculty of Medicine
University of British Columbia
Vancouver, British Columbia, Canada

RE: Dr. Rao Konduru's Publications   www.mydiabetescontrol.com

1. Permanent Diabetes Control
2. The Secret to Controlling Type 2 diabetes
3. Reversing Obesity
4. Reversing Sleep Apnea
5. Reversing Insomnia
6. Drinking Water Guide (www.DrinkingWaterGuide.com)

TO WHOM IT MAY CONCERN

Dr. Rao Konduru, PhD is a patient of mine who has suffered from chronic diabetes for most of his life; He also suffered from uncontrollable obesity, sleep apnea and chronic insomnia for the past 3 to 4 years. He has managed to reverse all of these conditions by taking non-pharmacological and science-based natural measures with great success. He has created 6 how-to user guides/books with regard to how he achieved this, and I recommend these books for anyone suffering from these conditions.

Sincerely,
Dr. Ali Ghahary, MD
Brentwood Medical Clinic
4567 Lougheed Hwy
Burnaby, British Columbia, Canada

RE: Permanent Diabetes Control (book)   www.mydiabetescontrol.com

Headline: Excellent Guide Regarding Diabetes

Dr. Rao Konduru's book, Permanent Diabetes Control, is a very useful guide and roadmap for anyone wishing to manage their diabetes well. It is an easy read and will be of great benefit. I intend to recommend this book to my diabetic patients.

Dr. Gary Almas, DPM-Podiatrist
4170 Fraser Street
Vancouver, British Columbia, Canada

RE: Permanent Diabetes Control (book)   www.mydiabetescontrol.com

We all know that food raises blood sugars, especially those big meals. We also know that exercise may reduce blood sugars. But Dr. Konduru teaches us how to put one and one together.

This book provides us with a method to accomplish a healthy lifestyle. Dr. Konduru learned it the hard way. After experiencing complications he decided to find the way his body likes to be treated. We, on the other hand, should learn from his experience and start implementing perfect blood sugar controls right now! Thank you, Dr. Rao Konduru, for providing the diabetic community with such a comprehensive book, on everything related to blood sugar control, including all up-to-date technology. I would recommend this book to every newly diagnosed and veteran diabetic!

Rabbi Hirsch Meisels
Moderator, FriendsWithDiabetes.Org
Spring Valley, New York, USA

RE: Permanent Diabetes Control (book)   www.mydiabetescontrol.com

Dr. Rao Konduru, in his book Permanent Diabetes Control, has made an outstanding contribution to the field of diabetes management. This is a book that will inspire its readers, whether diabetic or not, to make changes that will improve the quality of their lives forever. Through his own innovative experiments, Dr. Konduru has succeeded in developing a method of diabetes control that has allowed him, incredibly, to reduce his insulin dose by 60%, to reverse critical heart disease, thus avoiding bypass surgery, and to stabilize his blood glucose levels. In Permanent Diabetes Control, Dr. Konduru has carefully explained this method so that others may benefit from his revolutionary discovery. Join him in controlling your diabetes!

Ms. Ricki Ewings, BA, TT
Professional Freelance Writer and Editor
Member, Editors' Association of Canada
Hotline Co-Chair, EAC-BC
Vancouver, British Columbia, Canada

RE: Reversing Sleep Apnea (book)   www.reversingsleepapnea.com

Dear Rao,
I read your book this weekend and it is an impressively comprehensive and extremely well-documented review of the broad spectrum of therapies available to treat and help relieve sleep apnea. You are to be heartily congratulated on a finely-researched and very practical work that will be accessible and useful to a wide audience of readers. I wish you every success.

Best regards,
Mr. Martin R. Hoke
President
RhinoSystems, Inc.
Brooklyn Heights, OHIO-44131, USA

Other Publications of Rao Konduru, PhD

RE: Reversing Obesity (book)   www.ReversingSleepApnea.com/ebook2.html

This book "Reversing Obesity" will make you THIN in a matter of days by simply following the easy-to-understand rapid weight-loss instructions and the do-it-yourself recipes illustrated by Dr. RK. When the stubborn fat around his belly refused to melt away, Dr. RK took a wise decision. He very carefully jotted down all kinds of junk foods he had been eating here and there, every now and then. By exercising self-discipline and high willpower, he completely eliminated all those junk foods from his whole foods diet. Voila, the results were astounding! He started losing weight quickly as the stubborn fat melted away day-by-day right in front of his eyes. He explains how healthy whole foods are, and at the same time how harmful processed foods and refined foods are, and how to avoid them in order to achieve successful weight-loss results.

If you are obese or overweight, this book is a must-read to achieve rapid weight-loss results and to reverse many health disorders and diseases, including type 2 diabetes, sleep apnea and chronic insomnia.

  - Prime Publishing Co.
New Westminster, British Columbia, Canada

RE: Reversing Obesity (book)   www.ReversingSleepApnea.com/ebook2.html

This book "Reversing Obesity" isn't just any guide to miraculous weight loss. It is a compilation of hard-hitting facts, meticulous details and extraordinary results. It is the true and inspiring story of Dr. RK who succeeded in reversing his obesity permanently.

Healthy eating habits are necessary if one wants to lose weight and live well. In his book, Dr. RK teaches us simple, healthy and easy-to-make recipes using whole foods only. In addition, his weight-loss tips are extremely useful to implement the plan.

Dr. RK is a living example of a successful weight loss plan; a plan that helped him accomplish an absolute reversal of obstructive sleep apnea and chronic insomnia. After losing over 40 pounds of excess body weight more than a year back, he has maintained normal body weight until today, which is yet another achievement. This book has all the clues to not just rapid weight loss, but also on how to maintain normal weight after shedding off those extra pounds.

In my opinion, this book is the best thing that could ever happen to obese and overweight people. Only reading it could tell you why.

  - Ms. Muriel D'Souza, Advertising Copywriter, Vancouver, British Columbia, Canada
---

Other Publications of Rao Konduru, PhD

RE: Reversing Insomnia (book)   www.ReversingInsomnia.com

This book "Reversing Insomnia" is the simplest, and perhaps the safest way to cure chronic insomnia. Dr. RK has done all the spadework and leaves the rest of us to reap the benefits. All one has to do is read and follow the simple do-it-yourself instructions.

Hats off to Dr. RK and his impressive research. He figured how the master biological clock embedded in the brain works, and came up with an effortless and natural method to permanently cure chronic insomnia. He applied and tested his discovery on himself. It took him just 3 days to reverse his chronic insomnia after suffering from it for over 3 years.

After reading the entire book, I wholeheartedly believe it is the best cure for the sleep disorder. One, because it hardly takes time to cure the insomnia; two, because it has no side effects; and three, because sleeping pills are a complete waste of money.

It really works. So, just give it a try!

- Ms. Muriel D'Souza, Advertising Copywriter, Vancouver, British Columbia, Canada

RE: Reversing Insomnia (book)   www.ReversingInsomnia.com

At first we read "Reversing Obesity" another book by Dr. RK, and we found it better than the best books in the weight-loss industry. His recipe for the pre-workout meal "Egg White Omelet" is a major highlight. Anyone can lose weight by eating whole foods and by following the simple instructions for rapid weight loss method illustrated by Dr. RK.

After that we read his second book "Reversing Sleep Apnea" and we were blown away by its extremely impressive contents. Dr. RK convinces you beyond a shadow of a doubt that obstructive sleep apnea can be reversed simply and easily by losing weight. He has covered all the important therapies that a sleep apnea patient would ever need.

Then we read his third book "Reversing Insomnia" and his writing keeps getting more and more interesting. Dr. RK describes exactly where the planet Earth is located in our universe, and how it creates the daytime and nighttime by rotating on its own axis and by revolving around the sun. He divides the 24-hour master biological clock into two parts, one for the daytime and the other for the nighttime, and instructs the insomniacs what to do exactly as the day progresses and as the night progresses. By simply following his instructions, naturally, and without ever using sleeping pills, anyone can reset his/her master biological clock, and sleep like a baby within a few days. What a wonderful book!

- Prime Publishing Co.
New Westminster, British Columbia, Canada

REVIEWS: DRINKING WATER GUIDE by Rao Konduru, PhD

RE: Drinking Water Guide (book)   www.DrinkingWaterGuide.com

REVIEW: I was indeed thrilled to read through and learn the amazing descriptions about the formation of our Universe after the Big Bang, formation of stars, planets, galaxies, formation of our solar system, including our Sun and our planet Earth. Chapter 1, Chapter 13, Chapter 17, Chapter 18 & Chapter 19 contain the most valuable information. In a nutshell, this book teaches that we should avoid tap water, well water & bottled water, and drink only purified water that is either neutralized or slightly alkalized, and remineralized up to a TSD (Total Dissolved Solids) level of 200 ppm. The book teaches how to neutralize, slightly alkalize, fully alkalize and remineralize the purified water with sample experiments conducted at home. The book teaches healthy water-drinking habits, and gives recommendations at the end of each chapter. I greatly admire and recommend this highly researched, well-documented, and fully comprehensive guide on drinking water to every adult living on our planet Earth.   -- Prime Publishing Co., New Westminster, British Columbia, Canada.

Deanna Maio
5.0 out of 5 stars   Comprehensive Drinking Water Guide
Reviewed in the United States on February 17, 2020
Verified Purchase

NIKOLA TESLA said it all: "only a lunatic will drink unsterilized water". Very many people are still drinking unsterilized tap water and contaminated bottled water, jeopardizing their health, and developing strange diseases, and making many trips to hospitals and board-certified doctors. The tap water disaster incident that occurred in Flint, Michigan, USA in 2014 is a typical example of lead contamination that affected more than 100,000 residents.

This book describes about all kinds of drinking water available for human consumption, their defects, and appropriate "recommendations" in order to rectify those defects, and how to drink clean and healthy water in order to protect your health in the current day circumstances. This book Drinking Water Guide teaches many drinking water strategies:
(i) I must be wise and cautious all the time and should not take chances. I must not drink tap water, well water or bottled water of any kind, and make my own distilled water by purchasing and using a home distiller. Or, I must purchase RO water from a nearby supermarket, and I must always drink only purified water.
(ii) I would add very little Himalayan pink salt, Celtic sea salt or a few drops of ConcenTrace mineral drops to remineralize the purified water before drinking.
(iii) I would add a tiny bit of baking soda or a few drops of ConcenTrace mineral drops in order to improve the alkalinity and the presence of minerals in the purified water.
(iv) I would use pH strips or digital pH meter, monitor my drinking water pH, every now and then, and make sure that the purified water I drink is either neutralized (pH=7) or slightly alkalized (pH=7 to 7.5).
(v) I would use a TSD meter, and monitor the TDS level of my drinking water, and make sure that TDS level is always below 200 ppm. I will also research and find out the ideal TDS level that suits my body. I can do that by adjusting the tiny amount of Himalayan pink salt.

I am very grateful that I learned all the above-mentioned valuable information from this book "Drinking Water Guide". What an impressive book! I urge you to get this book without any hesitation.

Helpful   Comment   Report abuse

The Secret to Controlling Type 2 Diabetes
Addendum to "Permanent Diabetes Control" Book

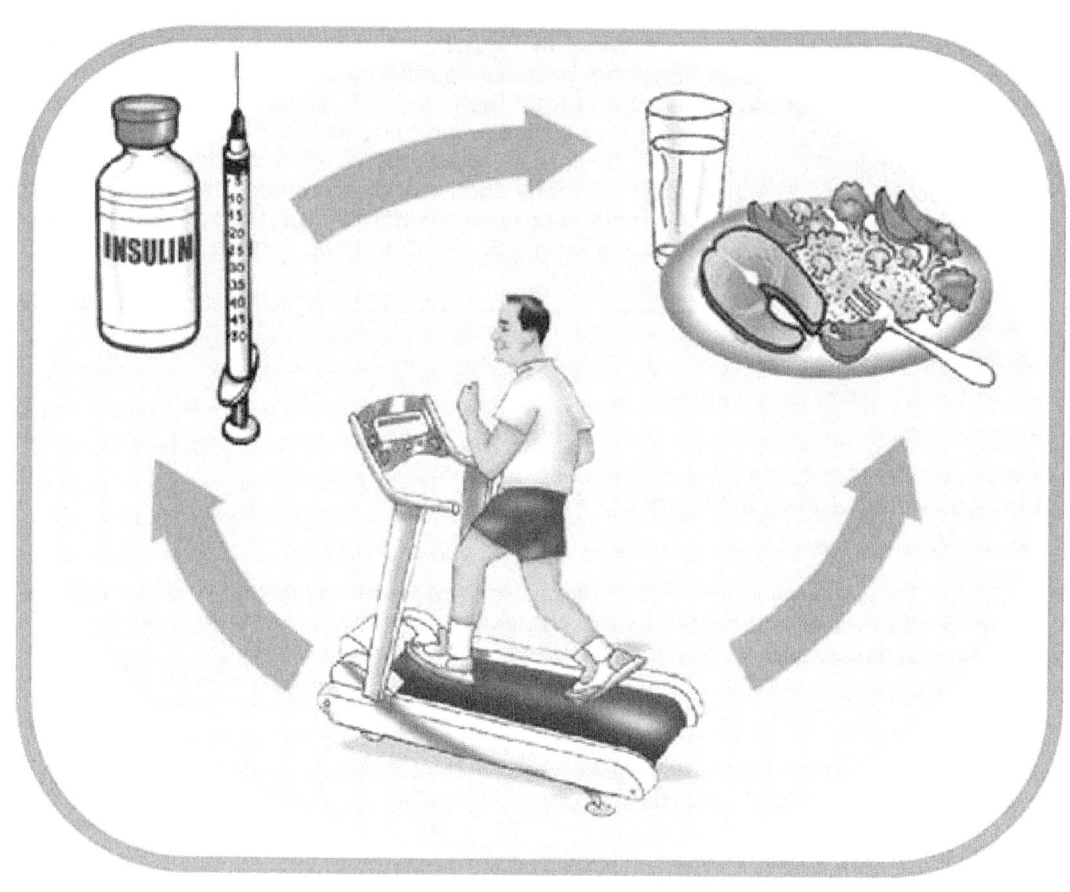

YOU WILL LEARN
- The Hidden Secret in The Hemoglobin A1c Chart!
- How to Find Out Your Daily Average Blood Glucose Level!
- How to Control Type 2 Diabetes With Diet & Exercise!
- How to Control Type 2 Diabetes With Diet, Oral Medication & Exercise!
- How to Control Type 2 Diabetes With Diet, Insulin Shots & Exercise!
- How to Control Type 1 Diabetes With Diet, Insulin Shots & Exercise!
- How to Lower Your Hemoglobin A1c to Perfectly Normal!
- How to Slash After-Meal Glucose Spikes & Achieve Normal A1c!

Rao Konduru, PhD

FOREWORD

Most diabetic people focus their attention on fasting blood-glucose levels in order to control diabetes, rather than on lowering after-meal glucose levels. Hemoglobin A1c is a parameter that directly reveals the degree of "diabetes control" during the preceding 90 days. Red blood cells live in the bloodstream 60 to 90 days. Every 90 days new red blood cells are born. Hemoglobin is a protein molecule that carries oxygen from the lungs to the body's cells wherever it is needed. While the blood circulates, depending on how high the blood glucose level is, a certain amount of glucose is attached to the hemoglobin to form A1c. So, by measuring the hemoglobin A1c level, it is possible to know the average blood glucose level and the degree to which it has been controlled over the preceding 90 days.

Blood glucose reaches its highest level immediately after a major meal consumption. The elevated glucose levels dominate in and largely contribute to establishing the average glucose level over 90 days. After-meal glucose levels therefore must be slashed and brought down to normal within 1 or 2 hours of after a major meal consumption, every day, in order to control and bring hemoglobin A1c close to its normal level or perfectly normal.

Pre-diabetes or borderline diabetes can be controlled with healthy diet and daily exercise. Mild or moderate Type 2 diabetes can be controlled with healthy diet, oral medication(s) and daily exercise. For severe Type 2 diabetes or Type 1 diabetes, oral medications do not work, and so it should be controlled with healthy diet, insulin shots and daily exercise.

If you are on insulin, be aware that the insulin dose must be minimized because too much insulin causes hypoglycemia and constricts arteries, leading to heart attack and coronary heart disease. Too much insulin also stimulates the brain so that a person feels hungry and eats more and causes the liver to manufacture fat in the belly. Too little insulin on the other hand would not be enough to cover the entire meal and to maintain normal blood glucose levels. An optimum insulin dose is therefore crucial. Insulin is synthesized in such a way that it acts more quickly and much more effectively with exercise. After-meal exercise, either treadmill or walking, should be introduced into the diabetes control plan in order to burn fat, lose calories and optimize both the insulin dose and insulin action. After-meal exercise minimizes the insulin dose and maximizes insulin action and prevents after-meal glucose levels from rising too high, thus keeping diabetes under tight control.

The research conducted by the author revealed the fact that consistent, serious and rigorous efforts towards lowering after-meal glucose levels over a period of 3 to 6 months gradually lowers the hemoglobin A1c level of a diabetic person to its normal level, even if the diabetes was poorly controlled in the past. Thereafter, continued efforts with a reasonable attention to insulin, food and exercise are necessary to tightly control diabetes.

The author of this book, having been diabetic for over 45 years, began to conduct diligent experiments 20 years ago to study the combined influence of insulin dose and after-meal exercise on after-meal blood glucose levels, and successfully lowered after-meal glucose levels continuously on a daily basis. For a selected major meal (supper/dinner), the Humalog insulin dose was cut by 50 to 60% through extensive research and optimization. The hemoglobin A1c level dropped from a very high-risk 12% to a stunning 6.5%, 6.0%, 5.5%, 5.0%, etc., and remained normal thereafter, indicating that the diabetes has been permanently controlled. Please refer to Chapter 3 & Chapter 4 to see the" Trial and Error Procedure: Diabetes Control", developed to determine the optimal insulin dose.

COPYRIGHT

Copyright © 2019-2020 and beyond by the Author.
All rights reserved under International and Pan-American Copyright laws.
This book is revised and rewritten in 2020.

Book Title:	The Secret to Controlling Type 2 Diabetes
Sub-Title:	Addendum to Permanent Diabetes Control
Author:	Rao Konduru, PhD (Also Called Dr. RK)
Publisher:	Prime Publishing Co.
Address:	720 – Sixth Street, Unit: 161
	New Westminster, BC, Canada, V3L-3C5
Website:	www.mydiabetescontrol.com
ISBN #:	ISBN 9780973112054

This book "Permanent Diabetes Control" has been properly registered under ISBN Number "ISBN 9780973112054" with the National Library of Canada Cataloguing in Publication, Ottawa, Ontario, Canada. The original manuscript has been submitted to the Legal Deposits, Library and Archives Canada, Ottawa, Ontario, Canada. All rights reserved!

WARNING: No part of this publication may be reproduced, distributed through the internet, or transmitted in any form or by any means, including photocopying for the purpose of redistributing the book among friends and loved ones. Reproduction of the ideas in this book without prior authorization constitutes a violation of the copyright and intellectual property laws.

DISCLAIMER

The author of the books titled "Permanent Diabetes Control" and "The Secret to Controlling Type 2 diabetes" assumes no liability or responsibility including, without limitation, incidental and consequential damages, personal injury or wrongful death resulting from the use of any treatment method presented in this book. The reader should take a training course in a local diabetes clinic (diabetes education center) on the insulin-dependant diabetes, and should learn all the aspects on how to inject rapid-acting insulin (such as Humalog), and how to exercise by running on a treadmill, biking, or regular walk in order to lower after-meal blood glucose level to perfectly normal. Without acquiring pertinent training and knowledge to use the treatment procedures illustrated in these books, it is warned not to act alone without supervision. The examples in this book mimic reality but were created for illustrative purposes. All contents in this book are for the educational purposes only and do not in any way represent the professional medical advice.

Dr. Rao Konduru's Publications	
1. Permanent Diabetes Control	www.mydiabetescontrol.com
2. The Secret to Controlling Type 2 Diabetes	www.mydiabetescontrol.com
3. Reversing Obesity	www.reversingosleepapnea.com/ebook2.html
4. Reversing Sleep Apnea	www.reversingsleepapnea.com
5. Reversing Insomnia	www.reversinginsomnia.com
6. Drinking Water Guide	www.drinkingwaterguide.com

The paperbacks (softcover book) and Kindle eBook are available for purchase on Amazon.com for US residents, and on Amazon.ca for Canadian residents.

TABLE OF CONTENTS

	Page
▶ Testimonials	i
▶ Foreword	1
▶ Copyright Page	2
▶ Table of Contents	3

	Page
● **CHAPTER 1: DIABETES FACTS & STATISTICS**	7
▶ Around the World	9
▶ In the USA	10
▶ In Canada	11
▶ Diabetes Statistics Resulted from Heart Disease	12
▶ Good News	12
◯ REFERENCES	13
● **CHAPTER 2: OVERVIEW OF DIABETES**	15
▶ How Glucose Builds Up In the Bloodstream?	17
▶ Diabetes and Pancreas	18
▶ Exocrine Function & Endocrine Function of Pancreas	19
▶ YouTube Videos About Pancreas	21
▶ The Production of Insulin in the Human Body	21
▶ Causes of Diabetes	21
▶ Symptoms of Diabetes	22
▶ Hyperglycemia Versus Hypoglycemia	22
▶ Reasons Why You Have Uncontrolled Diabetes	23
▶ Long Term Complications (Side Effects) of Diabetes	24
▶ Types of Diabetes	24
▶ Medical Check-Up and Diagnosis	26
▶ Self-Blood Glucose Monitoring Devices	27
▶ Continuous Glucose Monitoring Devices (Dexcom & FreeStyle)	28
▶ Routine Tests for Diabetics	29
▶ How Is Blood Glucose Level Expressed for Diabetes?	30
▶ Why Is the Glucose Conversion Factor 18?	30
▶ Normal Blood Glucose Levels and Normal & A1c Level	31
▶ An Example of Diabetes Control	31
◯ REFERENCES	32

	Page
● **CHAPTER 3: DIABETES CONTROL**	33
[A Very Important Chapter if You Are Diabetic]	
● **DIABETES CONTROL BASICS**	35
▶ Introduction to Diabetes Control	35
▶ Control Your Diabetes in 90 Days: Why 90 Days?	36
▶ Hemoglobin A1c & Hemoglobin A1c Chart Explained	36
▶ Normal Blood Glucose Levels & Normal Hemoglobin A1c Levels	38
▶ The Secret to Controlling Diabetes Successfully	38
▶ Example 1 & Example 2 to Understand the Secret	39
▶ Can the Hemoglobin A1c Be Determined At Home?	39
▶ How to Calculate Daily Average Blood Glucose Level?	41
▶ WHO CAN USE ORAL MEDICATIONS & WHO CAN USE INSULIN SHOTS?	43
● **HOW TO CONTROL DIABETES**	44
● **METHOD 1: Type 2 Diabetes Control**	45
With Healthy Diet & Exercise (No Medication)	
▶ Dietary Guidelines	45
▶ Physical Activity Stimulates the Insulin Production from Pancreas	46
▶ EXAMPLE 1: How to Control Type 2 Diabetes	46
With Healthy Diet, Daily Exercise & Self-Discipline!	
▶ Disadvantages of Method 1	48
● **METHOD 2: Type 2 Diabetes Control**	49
With Healthy Diet, Oral Medication & Exercise	
▶ Dietary Guidelines & Oral Medication	49
▶ Physical Activity Stimulates the Insulin Production from Pancreas	50
▶ EXAMPLE 2: How to Control Type 2 Diabetes	50
With Healthy Diet, Oral Medication, Daily Exercise & Self-Discipline!	
▶ Disadvantages of Method 2	52
● **METHOD 3: Type 2 Or Type 1 Diabetes Control**	55
With Healthy Diet, Insulin Shots & Exercise	
▶ Introduction	55
▶ Uncontrolled Diabetes Is Dangerous	55
▶ Insulin Is The Best Medication For Diabetes	55
▶ Important Note On Insulin	56
▶ Dietary Guidelines & Rapid-Acting Insulin	56
▶ Physical Activity Stimulates the Insulin Production from Pancreas	57
▶ Physical Activity Also Stimulates the Artificial Insulin Injected	58
▶ How Much Artificial Insulin Is to be Injected?	58
▶ Physical Activity Cuts Insulin Dose In Half	58
▶ Hands On Training Course In A Diabetes Clinic	59
▶ FIVE IMPORTANT PRECAUTIONS	59

	Page
▶ How to Achieve Normal A1c With Insulin Shots & Exercise?	62
● How to Enjoy High Carbohydrate Meals & Slash After-Meal Glucose Spikes?	62
● FIVE EXAMPLES DISCUSSED WITH DAILY DIABETES CONTROL ROUTINE	62
● Example 3, Example 4, Example 5, Example 6, Example 7	62
▶ Advantages of Method 3	73
▶ Disadvantages of Method 3	73
▶ Why Should the Insulin Dose Be Optimized?	74
▶ How to Optimize Insulin Dose by Trial & Error?	74
▶ Trial & Error Procedure: Simplified Approach	75
● For A Small Meal, Mid-Sized Meal & Large Meal	
▶ Trial & Error Procedure: Sophisticated Approach	77
▶ Trial & Error Procedure: Diabetes Control (Flow Sheet)	78
▶ Dr. RK's Diabetes Has Been Controlled Permanently	79
▶ Official Blood Test Results of the Controlled Diabetes	79
▶ CLOSING REMARKS	81
▶ WHAT IS PERMANENT DIABETES CONTROL?	81
◉ REFERENCES	81
◉ About the Author	89

CHAPTER 1 DIABETES FACTS & STATISTICS

TABLE OF CONTENTS

	Page
CHAPTER 1: DIABETES FACTS & STATISTICS	7
Around the World	9
In the USA	10
In Canada	11
Diabetes Statistics Resulted from Heart Disease	12
Good News	12
REFERENCES	13

AROUND THE WORLD

In 2017, the International Diabetes Federation (IDF) reported the following facts and statistics about people living with diabetes, after studying the prevalence and incidence of prediabetes or borderline diabetes, type 1 diabetes and type 2 diabetes, risk factors for complications, acute and long-term complications, deaths, and costs: [1]

- About 425 million adults are now living with diabetes around the world. By the year 2045, this number could rise to 619 million people. [1]

- More than 1,106,500 children have been living with type 1 diabetes. [1]

- Diabetes is a major public health problem that is approaching epidemic proportions globally. In general, 1 in 2 people with diabetes live undiagnosed. Type 2 diabetes is more rapidly growing, spreading and becoming an epidemic than type 1 diabetes. [1]

- Diabetes caused 4 million deaths during 2017 alone. [1]

- Diabetes caused at least $727 billion US dollars in health expenditure in 2017, which is 12% of total spending on adults. [1]

- The International Diabetes Federation (IDF) reported in 2005 in an article that type 2 diabetes affects a staggering 25 million European adults, adding another 6 million cases by the year 2025. IDF also reported that about 65 million European adults (one in 7 people) have impaired glucose tolerance syndrome due to which blood glucose levels jump too high after meals and remain normal or near-normal a few hours after meals or while fasting. The total healthcare expenditures for diabetes in Europe is estimated between 28 billion and 53 billion Euros per year. [1, 2]

- About 5 to 10% of diabetic people have type 1 diabetes. The remaining 90 to 95% of diabetic people have type 2 diabetes. About 90% of type 2 diabetic people are overweight or obese, as obesity and type 2 diabetes go hand in hand. A lot of type 2 diabetics are on insulin. [2, 4]

- About 3 to 20% of pregnant women develop gestational diabetes, depending on their risk factors. A diagnosis of gestational diabetes may increase the risk of developing diabetes later in life for both mother and child. [5]

- By the year 2025, developing countries such as India, China, Pakistan, Indonesia, Russia, Mexico, Brazil, Egypt, and Japan respectively are those most likely to be affected by diabetes in increased numbers as their people tend to adopt western lifestyles. [2, 3]

- Type 1 diabetes occurs equally in males and females. The World Health Organization project stated that type 1 diabetes is rare in most Asian, African and American Indian populations. But in Scandinavia, particularly in Sweden and Finland, type 1 diabetes rates are higher. The reason for this discrepancy is unknown. [2]

IN THE USA

● In 2017, The Centers for Disease Control and Prevention (CDC) released its diabetes statistics report with the following information: There are 30.3 million people with diabetes (9.4% of the US population) including 23.1 million people who are diagnosed, and 7.2 million people (23.8%) undiagnosed. The numbers for prediabetes indicate that 84.1 million adults (33.9% of the adult U.S. population) have prediabetes, including 23.1 million adults aged 65 years or older (the age group with highest rate). The estimated percentage of individuals with type 1 diabetes remains at 5% among those with diabetes. The statistics are also provided by age, gender, ethnicity, and for each state/territory so you can search for these specifics. [6]

● In 2015, The American Diabetes Association in 2015, published its diabetes statistics report with the following information: There are 30.3 million Americans (9.4% of the population) are living with diabetes. Approximately 1.25 million American children and adults have type 1 diabetes. Of those 30.3 Americans with diabetes, 23.1 million were diagnosed, and 7.2 million were undiagnosed. [7]

● Every year, another 1.5 million Americans are diagnosed with diabetes. [7]

● Diabetes was the seventh leading cause of death in the United States in 2015 based on the 79,535 death certificates. In 2015, diabetes was mentioned as a cause of death in a total of 252,806 certificates. Diabetes may be underreported as a cause of death. Studies have found that only about 35% to 40% of people with diabetes who died had diabetes listed anywhere on the death certificate and about 10% to 15% had it listed as the underlying cause of death. [7]

● In 2107, the total cost of diagnosed diabetes in the United States is $327 billion (USD), $237 billion was for direct medical costs, and $90 billion was in reduced productivity. [7]

● Despite the fact that in most cases most of the risk factors are preventable, the following staggering numbers occur in the USA: [2]

Kidney Disease: About 38,000 diabetic people face kidney failure every year, and more than 100,000 people are treated with a form of kidney disease. Over 50% of these cases are preventable. People with diabetes are 17 times more prone to kidney disease after being diabetic for 20 years or more.
Blindness and Eye Disease: As many as 12,000 to 24,000 diabetic people become blind every year while 90% of these cases could have been prevented.
Amputations: About 82,000 diabetic people undergo leg amputations every year while 85% of these cases could have been prevented.
Heart Disease and Stroke: Among the deaths of people with diabetes, more than 80% are due to heart disease and stroke though proper diabetes-care could have reduced 35% of deaths.
Gestational Diabetes: About 135,000 expectant mothers are diagnosed with gestational diabetes every year, and the babies thus born experience an increased risk of serious complications in the future. Appropriate care during pregnancy could significantly reduce such risk.
Flu and Pneumonia: Between 10,000 and 30,000 diabetic people die every year due to complications related to flu and pneumonia. People with diabetes are three times more likely to die from flu and pneumonia than those without diabetes.

IN CANADA

- In Canada, over 3 million people live with and have diabetes, that's just over 9% of our total population. Unfortunately, that number is expected to rise. Diabetes Canada estimates that by the year 2025, a staggering 5 million people (12% of the population) will have diabetes. [8]

- Currently, there are 11 million Canadians living with prediabetes or borderline diabetes. That means that almost one in three people in Canada are affected by this condition. Prediabetes is a condition in which blood glucose levels are higher than normal, but haven't reached the level required for a diagnosis of type 2 diabetes. If prediabetes is undiagnosed or untreated, it can eventually lead to type 2 diabetes. [8]

- Statistics Canada in 2017 reported that 7.3% of Canadians aged 12 and older (roughly 2.3 million people) were diagnosed with diabetes. Between 2016 and 2017, the proportion of males who reported being diagnosed with diabetes increased from 7.6% in 2016 to 8.4% in 2017. The proportion of females remained consistent between the two years. [9]

- Canadians with type 1 diabetes have been living with their diagnosis for an average of 20.2 years, compared to 12.2 years for type 2 diabetes. Overall, males (8.4%) were more likely than females (6.3%) to report that they had diabetes. Diabetes increased with age for males, with the highest prevalence among those 75 years and older. The percentage of females reporting diabetes increased with age up to the age of 64, the prevalence did not increase significantly for those aged 75 and older. [9]

- Canadian adults, older than 18, who were either overweight or obese were more likely than those who were classified as having a normal weight to report that they had been diagnosed with diabetes. The prevalence of diabetes among obese Canadians was 13.7% in 2017, compared with 6.8% among overweight Canadians and 3.6% among those classified as having a normal weight. [9]

DIABETES STATISTICS RESULTED FROM HEART DISEASE [2]

Believe it or not, the following staggering information is true:

● Diabetes (living with high blood glucose levels) is the major reason of heart disease.

● More than 80 percent of people with diabetes die from some form of heart or blood vessel disease.

● The World Health Organization (WHO), the International Society and Federation of Cardiology (ISFC) and the United Nations Educational, Scientific and Cultural Organization (UNESCO) jointly reported in a press release in 1997 that cardiovascular diseases kill more than any other disease around the world. Every year, an estimated 15 million deaths are reported, which is about 30% of total deaths around the world, and many more millions of people are disabled due to heart and blood vessel diseases.

● Cardiovascular disease has been the number one killer in the USA since 1900 (heart disease being the first leading cause of death and stroke being the 3rd leading cause of death).

● About 61 million Americans (about one-fourth of the population) live with the complications of heart disease and stroke. In 2001, the cost for all cardiovascular diseases in the USA alone was $300 billion.

● Every 33 seconds, a person dies from cardiovascular disease in the USA alone.

● Every 34 seconds, a person dies from a form of heart disease in the USA alone.

● Every day, more than 2500 Americans die from heart disease.

● Every year, more than 250,000 people die of heart attack in the USA before they reach a nearby hospital.

● In 1991, 923,000 Americans died from heart and blood vessel diseases.

● Also, in countries like Russia, Romania, Bulgaria, Hungary, Bulgaria, Czechoslovakia and Poland, heart disease contributes to the highest number of deaths. The lowest death rates of heart disease were in Japan, France, Spain, Switzerland and Canada.

GOOD NEWS
● However, the good news is that many celebrities, famous athletes, Hollywood stars, wealthy people, politicians and highly qualified professionals of all types educational background, including doctors, engineers, lawyers, businessmen and businesswomen have experienced type 1 or type 2 diabetes, treated themselves successfully with proper knowledge and care and lived long and healthy. They demonstrated that they have willpower (knowledge is power) to fight and control diabetes.

● Controlling diabetes which is the only subject matter of this book as a matter of fact is a very interesting and enjoyable task. Please refer to Chapter 3 and Chapter 4, and learn how to control your diabetes permanently.

REFERENCES

1. Diabetes Facts & Figures (Statistics) by International Diabetes Federation (IDF)
https://www.idf.org/aboutdiabetes/what-is-diabetes/facts-figures.html

2. Permanent Diabetes Control (Book), Subtitle: The Complete Guide to Living Like A Normal Person Forever, Authored by Rao Konduru, MS, PhD, Reviewed and Endorsed by Dr. Marshal Dahl, MD, PhD., Endocrinologist, Faculty of Medicine, University of British Columbia, Vancouver, British Columbia, Canada, First Published in 2003.
www.mydiabetescontrol.com

3. Eve Gehling, M.Ed, The Family & Friends' Guide to Diabetes, John Wiley & Sons, New York, NY, USA, page 39, 2000.

4. Diabetes: Facts, Statistics, and You by Healthline.
https://www.healthline.com/health/diabetes/facts-statistics-infographic#1

5. What is diabetes? Types of Diabetes by Canadian Diabetes Association, 2019.
https://www.diabetes.ca/diabetes-basics/what-is-diabetes

6. The 2017 National Diabetes Statistics by American Association of Diabetes Educators by by Karen Kemmis, PT, DPT, MS, CDE, FAADE, Posted on July 26, 2017.
https://www.diabeteseducator.org/news/aade-blog/aade-blog-details/karen-kemmis-pt-dpt-ms-cde-faade/2017/07/26/the-2017-national-diabetes-statistics-report-is-here

7. Diabetes Statistics by American Diabetes Association, The Data Collected in 2015.
http://www.diabetes.org/diabetes-basics/statistics/
https://www.diabetes.org/resources/statistics/statistics-about-diabetes

8. Living Well With Diabetes by Diabetes Care Community.
https://www.diabetescarecommunity.ca/living-well-with-diabetes-articles/managing-diabetes-canada/

9. Diabetes-2017, Heath Fact Sheets by Statistics Canada.
https://www150.statcan.gc.ca/n1/pub/82-625-x/2018001/article/54982-eng.htm

CHAPTER 2 OVERVIEW OF DIABETES

TABLE OF CONTENTS

	Page
CHAPTER 2: OVERVIEW OF DIABETES	15
How Glucose Builds Up In the Bloodstream?	17
Diabetes and Pancreas	18
Exocrine Function & Endocrine Function of Pancreas	19
YouTube Videos About Pancreas	21
The Production of Insulin in the Human Body	21
Causes of Diabetes	21
Symptoms of Diabetes	22
Hyperglycemia Versus Hypoglycemia	22
Reasons Why You Have Uncontrolled Diabetes	23
Long Term Complications (Side Effects) of Diabetes	24
Types of Diabetes	24
Medical Check-Up and Diagnosis	26
Self-Blood Glucose Monitoring Devices	27
Continuous Glucose Monitoring Devices (Dexcom & FreeStyle)	28
Routine Tests for Diabetics	29
How Is Blood Glucose Level Expressed for Diabetes?	30
Why Is the Glucose Conversion Factor 18?	30
Normal Blood Glucose Levels and Normal & A1c Level	31
An Example of Diabetes Control	31
REFERENCES	32

ARE YOU DIABETIC?
UNDERSTAND HOW GLUCOSE BUILDS UP IN THE BLOODSTREAM! [1]

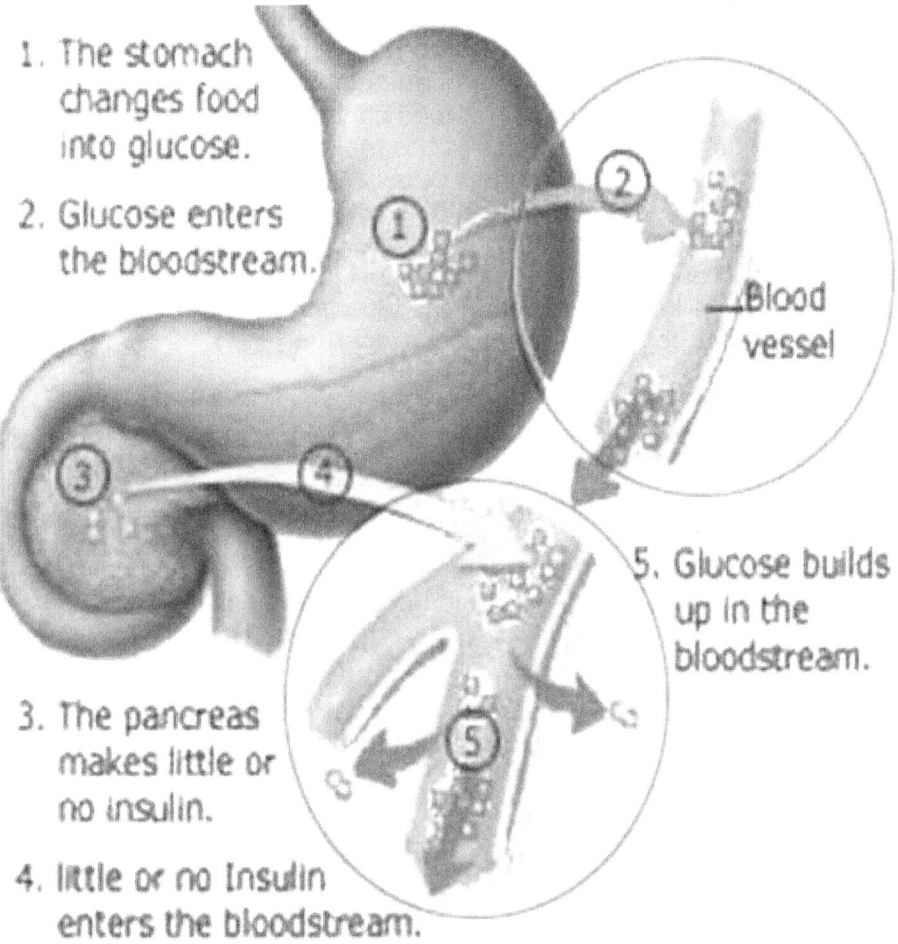

Figure 2.1 Glucose buildup in the blood stream.

1. The stomach changes food into glucose immediately after digestion.
2. Glucose enters the blood stream.
3. The pancreas makes little or no insulin if you are diabetic.
   Insulin is essential for aiding glucose transport into the trillions of body's cells.
   Insulin drives glucose molecules through the bloodstream.
4. Little or no insulin enters the bloodstream if you are diabetic.
5. Glucose builds up in the bloodstream because of the lack of insulin flow, and so you will be living with high blood glucose levels throughout the day, or your body's cells are unable to absorb the glucose due a kind of metabolic disorder, and therefore will be diagnosed with diabetes.

⦿ Diabetes over time damages essential components in your body, mostly your blood vessels in all parts of your body, arteries, nerves, and other parts. The long-term side effects or complications of uncontrolled diabetes can be very serious, and some of them could eventually be fatal. So take action immediately if you have diabetes!

DIABETES AND PANCREAS [1]

Diabetes Mellitus means "sweet urine" being siphoned through the urinary system out of the body. Diabetes is a Greek word meaning "to siphon", and Mellitus is a Latin word meaning "honey". Diabetes, when uncontrolled, is a chronic and fatal condition or disease developed due to the pancreatic deficiency in producing an adequate amount of insulin or due to the body's inability to properly utilize insulin. The food consumed is broken down by digestive juices into a simple sugar called glucose which is the main source of energy. The insulin drives glucose via the bloodstream into the body's cells to be used as energy. When the beta cells of the pancreas are destroyed and produce little or no insulin, the glucose builds up in the bloodstream, leading to diabetes. Also, when the body's cells become unable to respond to insulin secretion due to a a kind of metabolic disorder, diabetes develops. When the glucose level is markedly elevated in the bloodstream, the glucose overflows into the urine thus losing the body's main source of energy.

When the person's glucose levels in the bloodstream are no longer normal and unusually high, the person is diagnosed with diabetes or the person is said to be diabetic. The good news is that diabetes is not contagious and is fully controllable.

The pancreas of the human body as shown in the figure below is situated on the left side of the body underneath the stomach just beneath the liver. The pancreas is a soft, pinkish-gray colored banana-shaped gland of about 15 to 25 cm long. The pancreas is connected to the upper part of the small intestine by means of a duct.

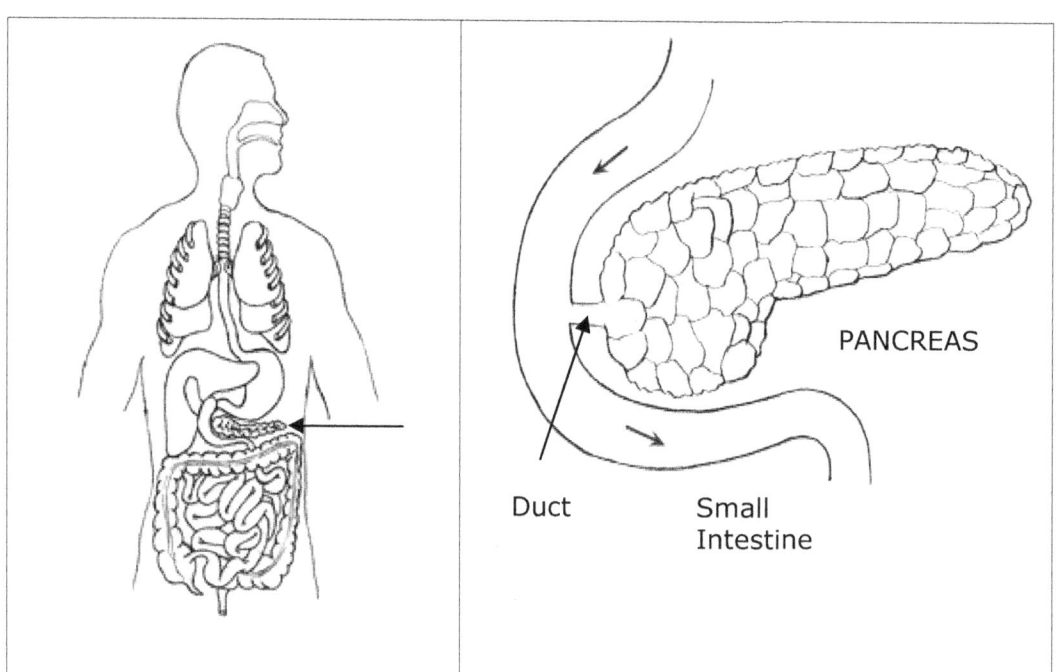

Figure 2.2 Picture of the human pancreas.

The Human Pancreas Serves Two Major Functions: [1]
(i) Exocrine Function (to produce digestive juices)
(ii) Endocrine Function (to produce insulin and glucagon)

In 1869, Dr. Paul Langerhans first identified that endocrine cells under low power magnification appear to be islands (islets) and since then they were named "Islets of Langerhans." Exocrine cells do not secrete any product into the bloodstream while endocrine cells do. A normal pancreas contains about 1 million cells, 1 to 2% of which are islets of Langerhans, very small bits of tissue at the tail end of the pancreas, embedded in exocrine pancreatic acinar tissue.

Each islet of Langerhans is made up of four different cells: alpha cells to secrete glucagon, beta cells to secrete insulin, gamma cells to secrete pancreatic polypeptide and delta cells to secrete somatostatin. The amazing beta cells are capable of sensing and measuring the blood glucose level within seconds and secrete an adequate amount of already stored insulin instantly.

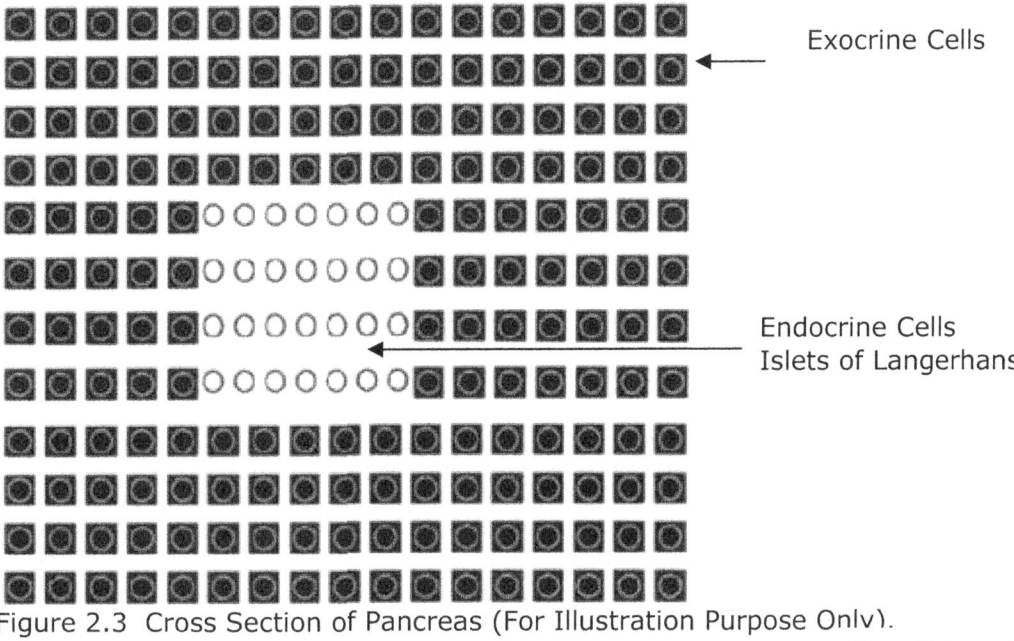

Figure 2.3 Cross Section of Pancreas (For Illustration Purpose Only).

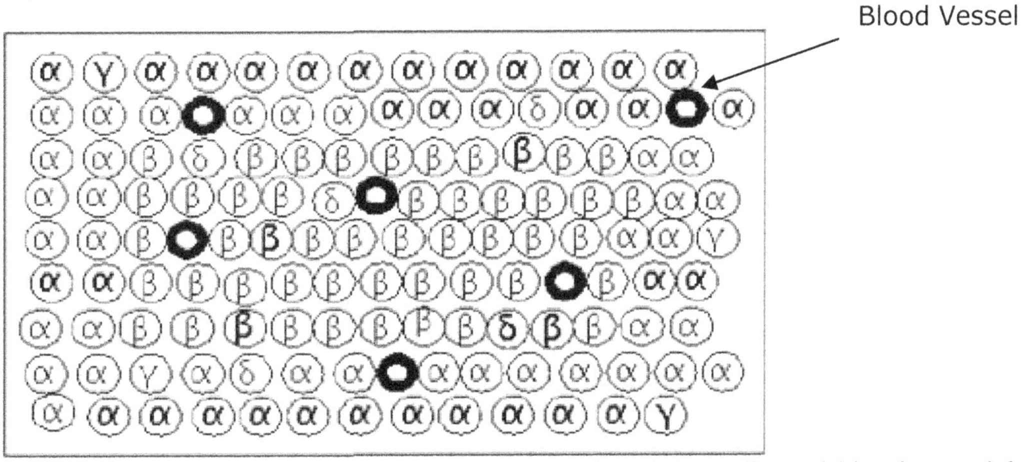

Figure 2.4 ISLET OF LANGERHANS (Beta cells, Alpha cells and blood vessels).

The Exocrine function of the pancreas is to produce a digestive alkaline juice that is enriched with about 15 different enzymes. This digestive juice passes through a duct as shown in Figure 1.1 and mixes with finely chewed and crushed food that is coming through the stomach and enters into the small intestine for further digestion. These enzymes break down different types of food into small particles in order to promote digestion. Some enzymes digest protein, some digest fat and others digest carbohydrate. The liver receives all sugars from the intestine walls and converts them into glucose—the body's main source of energy. The glucose is then distributed via the bloodstream to all cells of the body. When the exocrine function fails, enzymes lack and indigestion develops.

The Endocrine function of the pancreas is to control and regulate glucose level in the bloodstream by secreting the appropriate amount of insulin. The function of the islets of Langerhans is to produce two important hormones called insulin and glucagon. Beta cells produce insulin while alpha cells produce glucagon. Glucagon stimulates the cells of liver, muscle and kidney tissue to break down the already stored glycogen. Glycogen is the long chains of glucose stored in the liver, muscles and kidneys for future use. Whenever there is excess glucose in the bloodstream from digested food, the excess glucose is converted into glycogen. As shown in Figure 2.3, there are enough blood vessel inlets to receive either insulin or glucagon. Insulin and glucagon act mutually against each other to maintain normal glucose levels in the bloodstream. Whenever food is consumed, glucose from digested food is absorbed by the small intestine walls and is released into the bloodstream and blood glucose levels rise. Higher glucose levels stimulate the beta cells, which in turn secrete insulin into the bloodstream, and at the same time inhibit glucagon release from pancreatic alpha cells. Thus the insulin level gradually rises in the bloodstream and acts on the liver, fat and muscle cells to absorb the incoming molecules of glucose, amino acids and fatty acids. This action prevents the glucose level from rising too high. After a few hours of meal consumption or while fasting, the glucose level begins to drop. At this particular time, the pancreatic alpha cells secrete glucagon, which stimulates the liver to break down glycogen and release glucose. The glucose level in the bloodstream therefore begins to rise automatically. This counter-action of glucagon against insulin prevents the glucose levels from falling too low for a non-diabetic person. When the food is consumed next time during the day, the higher amounts of glucose from digested food again enters the bloodstream, beta cells get stimulated and the insulin secretion controls the glucose level, and so on. This is called the principle of "negative feedback control". This is how the healthy pancreas of a non-diabetic person maintains automatic counter-balance between the actions of insulin and glucagon and normal glucose levels all the time. Any defect caused by the poor functioning of the pancreas contributes to a lack of insulin supply or metabolic disorder due to which the body's cells become unable to utilize the insulin secretion properly, and the end result is a life-threatening build up of elevated glucose levels in the bloodstream causing a chronic and possibly fatal disease called ***"diabetes mellitus."***

The amazing counter-action between β-Cells and α-Cells situated in the islets of Langerhans is responsible to maintain normal blood glucose levels for healthy non-diabetic people. β-Cells produce insulin while α-Cells produce glucagon.

$$\beta\text{-Cells} \longrightarrow \text{Insulin}$$
$$\text{Glucagon} \longleftarrow \alpha\text{-Cells}$$

YouTube Videos About Pancreas

Watch the following YouTube videos to better understand the function of pancreas of the human body. [3, 4]

3. YouTube Video, Title: What is Pancreas?, Published by Rahul Azad, Aug 24, 2009
https://www.youtube.com/watch?v=1l2GTGEwZOY&feature=youtu.be
4. YouTube Video, Title: How the Body Works: The Pancreas, Published by Daniel Izzo, Aug 3, 2017
https://www.youtube.com/watch?v=j5WF8wUFNkI&feature=youtu.be

THE PRODUCTION OF INSULIN IN THE HUMAN BODY [1]

The production of insulin in the beta cells of a non-diabetic person is a two-step process. Beta cells first produce preproinsulin which is cleaved to produce pro-insulin, which is further cleaved to produce equal amounts of insulin and C-peptide. The insulin thus produced in beta cells has a half-life of about four minutes in the bloodstream (Half-life means the time required to decay one-half of the insulin produced). C-peptide lasts about 30 minutes.

The amazing beta cells of the pancreas sense and measure blood glucose within seconds and secrete the appropriate amount of insulin into the bloodstream in order to maintain normal glucose level all the time.

A VERY IMPORTANT NOTE: A healthy non-diabetic person's pancreas stores about 200 units of insulin, measures blood glucose level 500 times a day, and automatically secretes the appropriate amount of insulin into the bloodstream in order to maintain normal blood glucose level throughout the day. If you are diagnosed with diabetes, you should monitor and adjust insulin supply as frequently as possible and take action to adjust the insulin flow. But the problem is that the most diabetic people don't monitor even 5 times a day.

In a diabetic person, due to pancreatic deficiency, the body does not monitor glucose levels as adequately as needed nor does it adjust or supply sufficient insulin in the bloodstream to maintain normal glucose levels. So a diabetic person is required to monitor glucose levels as frequently as possible with an intention to control them. Only in this way, can diabetes be self-controlled.

CAUSES OF DIABETES [1]

- Heredity is the major reason. The defects associated with the function of the pancreas are duplicated from parents to children.
- Destruction of body's immune system leads to pancreatic dysfunction.
- Viruses could play a role in damaging the pancreas causing diabetes.
- Obesity can cause insulin resistance leading to diabetes.
- Some medications cause steroid-induced diabetes.
- Women who do not get enough to eat during first three months of their pregnancies give birth to babies who have short legs and who later develop Type 2 diabetes.
- Pregnant women could develop diabetes during the stress of pregnancy, and then both the mother and child could develop diabetes within 15 years after the pregnancy.

SYMPTOMS OF DIABETES [1, 5]

The following are the symptoms of diabetes a person experiences during and after the development of prediabetes or diabetes. A person should get tested for diabetes when experiences any of the following symptoms, and take appropriate action to treat diabetes.

- Frequent urination & Increased thirst,
- Fatigue or tiredness due to loss of glucose through urine,
- Disorientation or Irritability,
- Unexplained weight loss or weight gain,
- Extreme hunger,
- Presence of ketones in the urine (ketones are a byproduct of the breakdown of muscle and fat that happens when there is not enough insulin available in blood vessels),
- Blurred vision due to low blood sugars,
- Frequent infections on gums, skin, feet and vaginal infections, and slow healing from infections.

HYPERGLYCEMIA VERSUS HYPOGLYCEMIA [1]

Hyperglycemia and hypoglycemia are two extreme symptoms of diabetes. All people with type 1, type 2 and gestational diabetes may experience both symptoms of hyperglycemia and hypoglycemia. The following table shows the major differences between them.

Table 2.1 Hyperglycemia versus hypoglycemia.

HYPERGLYCEMIA	HYPOGLYCEMIA
Symptoms	**Symptoms**
Extreme thirst, urination, weakness, loss of appetite, nausea, vomiting.	Nervousness, sweating, hunger, blurred vision, imbalance.
Indications	**Indications**
High levels of glucose in blood and urine (over 13 mmol/L or 230 mg/dL).	Low levels of glucose in blood (below 4 mmol/L or 72 mg/dL).
Too little insulin in the blood.	Too much insulin in the blood.
Treatment	**Treatment**
Monitor glucose in the blood.	Monitor glucose in the blood.
Monitor glucose and ketones in urine.	Eat sugar, candy, orange juice,
Drink sugar-free fluids or water.	coke, etc. to raise glucose levels.
Exercise to bring glucose level down.	Inject glucagon if unconscious.
Inject insulin or take pill to treat hyper.	

REASONS WHY YOU HAVE UNCONTROLLED DIABETES [10]

- If your hemoglobin A1c result from a laboratory blood test is found to be over 7% or 0.07, your diabetes is said to be uncontrolled. Most diabetics don't know how to control diabetes, and live with elevated A1c level for decades despite trying hard a variety of oral medications, despite the daily insulin injections, and many trips to diabetes specialists.

- You are not monitoring enough and not researching enough to understand your elevated after-meal glucose spikes, and not supplementing your body with enough artificial insulin as you lack fine tuning skills.

- Did you know a healthy non-diabetic person's pancreas monitors blood glucose level 500 times a day, and automatically adjusts the insulin secretion to keep up the normal blood glucose levels throughout the day? This is called the "fine-tuning" skill of the pancreas. A diabetic person should monitor as many times as possible, and supplement insulin, to keep up the normal blood glucose levels. If you are a beginner in controlling your diabetes, you should monitor 10 times a day (5 fasting glucose levels and 5 after meal glucose levels), and analyse the data to better understand how your blood glucose levels are being fluctuated and how to control them. If you don't do that, your diabetes will remain uncontrolled.

- Even the doctors, endocrinologists and board-certified specialists are not equipped with the appropriate knowledge and training skills to transmit the real concept of controlling diabetes to their patients' minds, except leaving their patients in a dilemma of uncontrolled diabetes.

- The doctors don't teach their patients how to understand the hemoglobin A1c chart with clear concept. As a matter of fact, the secret to controlling diabetes lies in understanding the hemoglobin chart. And nobody ever told you about it, and nobody ever taught you that secret!

- You have been on oral medications for a long time, and did not think about switching to insulin shots because nobody convinced you that insulin is the best medicine to treat diabetes.

- Your hemoglobin A1c is not normal because you are not injecting enough insulin at appropriate times except some scheduled doses recommended by your doctor or nurse, and you are not exercising enough to lower after-meal spikes. And your doctors have been giving you full freedom to live like the way you want with unhealthy lifestyle.

- You are partying too much and eating too much with your family and friends every now and then. Your temptation to eat something delicious would lead to loss of control on dietary guidelines, causing you to overeat delicious foods that are made from processed and refined foods. Your unhealthy eating habits contribute to high blood glucose levels throughout the day, which further contribute to elevated A1c level.

- Most important of all of the above, you lack self-efficacy, self-discipline, motivation, and willpower to fight and control your diabetes and achieve normal hemoglobin A1c level.

LONG-TERM COMPLICATIONS (SIDE-EFFECTS) OF DIABETES
UNCONTROLLED DIABETES IS DANGEROUS! [1, 5]

Do not simply rely on oral medications, waste year after year, and live with uncontrolled diabetes. Living with uncontrolled diabetes, and neglecting your health by inadequately managing your chronic diabetes means you are living with high glucose levels in the bloodstream, and high levels of hemoglobin A1c. At elevated blood glucose levels over a long time, the glucose sticks to the surface of the cells and it is then converted into a poison called "sorbitol", which damages the body's cells and blood vessels, leading to long-term side effects such as:

- High cholesterols (total cholesterol & LDL cholesterol) and high blood pressure,
- Heart attack, heart failure, coronary heart disease, stroke,
- Hardening of arteries or what is known as atherosclerosis,
- Peripheral artery disease (PAD), narrowing of arteries,
- Painful neuropathy (nerve damage and poor blood flow),
- Burning foot syndrome, numbness in feet and knees, intermittent claudication,
- Amputation (due to nerve damage in the feet),
- Kidney disease, kidney damage, loss of kidney,
- Erectile dysfunction (ED) and/or Impotence,
- Cataracts, blurred vision, retinopathy, blindness,
- Deafness (hearing impairment),
- Diseases of the small blood vessels in the eyes, kidneys, legs and nerves,
- Gum disease and bone loss (dental problems),
- Bladder and prostate problems,
- Skin diseases (bacterial and fungal infections),
- Dementia such as Alzheimer's disease,
- Depression develops over time if diabetes is left untreated,
- and many other strange problems and complications.

If your hemoglobin A1c from a blood test is more than 7%, your diabetes in uncontrolled, so take action immediately! When the after-meal blood glucose spike is too high after eating and remain elevated for more than two hours, this presents a significant mortality risk factor, and the person should switch to insulin shots, and should learn how to slash after meal spikes by incorporating exercise.

Learn how to control your diabetes permanently by reading through this book thoroughly.

TYPES OF DIABETES (Brief Description)

In Short, the Following are the Types of Diabetes: [2]

Prediabetes or Borderline Diabetes: Blood glucose levels are higher than what's considered normal, but not high enough to qualify as diabetes disease.
Type 1 diabetes: The pancreas produces no insulin, and so you need to inject insulin.
Type 2 diabetes: The pancreas doesn't make enough insulin or your body can't use it effectively, thereby developing type 2 diabetes.
Gestational Diabetes: Expectant or pregnant women are unable to make and use all of the insulin they need during pregnancy.

TYPES OF DIABETES (Elaborated Description) [1]

There are 3 types of diabetes:
(i) Type 1 Diabetes,
(ii) Type 2 Diabetes, and
(iii) Gestational Diabetes

Type 1 Diabetes Mellitus or insulin-dependent diabetes mellitus or adult diabetes, also called juvenile diabetes, is developed when the pancreas produces little or no insulin because the beta cells of the pancreas may have been totally damaged or destroyed. Type 1 diabetes is developed mostly in infants, children and young adults under the age 30 years. About 10% to 15% of the diabetics belong to the type 1 group. Insulin shots are required to treat type 1 diabetes.

Type 2 Diabetes or non-insulin dependent diabetes, also called adult-onset diabetes, is developed when the pancreas produces insufficient insulin because the beta cells of the pancreas may have been partly damaged. Even if the pancreas produces insulin well, the body tissues do not respond adequately to the insulin, becoming resistant to insulin. This is called insulin resistance. Insulin resistance is the underlying problem with type 2 diabetic people. About 85% to 90% of diabetics belong to type 2. Type 2 diabetics take oral medications. Some type 2 diabetics take insulin shots when the pills don't work. A lot of type 2 diabetics are now getting used to insulin shots to quickly offset the elevated glucose levels. Diabetes can be more precisely controlled with insulin as it acts much more effectively than pills.

Gestational Diabetes is developed temporarily in women during pregnancy mostly during the last three months. All pregnant women must be checked for diabetes several times during pregnancy. If diagnosed with gestational diabetes, nearly 40% of women usually develop type 2 diabetes later in life within 15 years. A non-diabetic woman, diagnosed with diabetes during pregnancy, should control diabetes to its fullest extent to protect herself and for the sake of a healthy child. A diabetic woman who is pregnant needs to take extra care. A pregnant woman is said to be diagnosed with gestational diabetes when she is tested positive for any two of the following:

   a. A fasting plasma glucose level of more than 5.8 mmol/L or 105 mg/dL.
   b. One-hour after-meal level of more than 10.6 mmol/L or190 mg/dL.
   c. Two-hour after-meal level of more than 9.2 mmol/L or 165 mg/dL.
   d. Three-hour after-meal level of more than 8.1 mmol/L or 145 mg/dL.

MEDICAL CHECK-UP AND DIAGNOSIS [1, 6]

If the pancreas of a person does not function properly, firstly the person experiences indigestion problem because of the lack of enzymes. Poor absorption of food causes weight loss and diarrhea. Secondly, there would be not enough insulin production, resulting in frequent urination, loss of glucose through urine, increased thirst and weight loss. In order to diagnose a person with diabetes, the following tests are performed:

- **The Chemcard Glucose Test:** It is a simple FDA approved screening test for diabetes, being used to quickly identify an abnormally high fasting plasma glucose level. It is a 3-minute test that requires a single drop of blood from a fingerstick. This unit is for both home use and in doctors' offices. This test kit does not require any laboratory analysis and is still 94 to 99.95% accurate. When a person approaches a physician with these symptoms of frequent urination and increased thirst, the physician readily suspects that the problem is related to diabetes. After a physical examination, and after obtaining information regarding symptoms and family history, the physician could instantly test the urine and blood from a fingerstick, and from these test results, the physician could tentatively determine if the person is diabetic or not.

- **The Oral Glucose Tolerance Test**: It is an important test in which the physician asks the patient to come back early in the morning after fasting for 10 hours but not greater than 16 hours. The patient is asked to consume 75 grams of glucose (dissolved in purified water), and the glucose levels are then monitored at intervals of 15 minutes or 30 minutes for a period of 2 to 3 hours. A non-diabetic person's glucose level gradually drops to normal in 2 hours (under 7.8 mmol/L or 140 mg/dL), whereas a diabetic person's glucose levels remain significantly higher (more than 11.1 mmol/L or 200 mg/dL) and the levels do not drop to normal until and after 6 hours, confirming that the person has diabetes.

- **Random Blood Glucose Test:** Regardless of when you last ate, a blood sample showing that your blood sugar level is 200 mg/dL (11.1 mmol/L) or higher suggests diabetes, especially if you also have signs and symptoms of diabetes, such as frequent urination and extreme thirst.
- **Fasting Blood Glucose Test.** A blood sample is taken after an overnight fast. A reading of less than 5.6 mmol/L or 100 mg/dL is normal. A level from 5.6 to 6.9 mmol/L or 100 to 125 mg/dL is considered prediabetes. If your fasting blood glucose level is more than 7 mmol/L or 126 mg/dL on two separate tests, you will be diagnosed with diabetes.
- **More Tests:** The physician could conduct more useful tests. The level of amylase in the blood could reveal inflammation of the pancreas. An excess quantity of fat present in the blood sample indicates that the pancreas is not producing enough enzymes. An ultrasound scan test gives pictures of the pancreas gland to see any physical damage. The physician, by carefully inserting a needle, collects a small piece of pancreas gland and sends it to a pathologist for further examination. There are also more tests available such as CT Scan, endoscopic retrograde cholangiopancreatography (ERCP) to see if the pancreas is damaged.

- **C-peptide Test:** It is also important to find out if the pancreas is producing any insulin or not. By measuring the amount of C-peptide present in the blood, it is possible to determine the amount of insulin produced by the pancreas. Type 1 diabetic people have decreased levels of insulin and C-peptide while type 2 diabetic people have normal or increased levels of C-peptide.

- **Hemoglobin A1c Test:** Ultimately, a hemoglobin A1c blood test would precisely reveal the average blood glucose level of a person over the preceding 90 days, based on which a physician can easily understand if the patient being tested is diabetic or non-diabetic, and take appropriate steps if the patient is diagnosed with diabetes.

SELF-BLOOD GLUCOSE MONITORING DEVICES [1]

If you are diagnosed with diabetes, it is time to purchase a self-blood glucose monitoring device for home use, learn how to use it, and start monitoring and recording your daily blood glucose levels throughout the day (not just fasting glucose level in the morning). The best advice is that a diabetic patient must monitor at least 3 fasting blood glucose levels and 3 after meal blood glucose levels, meaning 6 times a day. The more frequently you monitor, the better you diabetes control could be. Whenever you monitor, if the blood glucose level is too high or not normal, you must take action by exercising or taking a medication (either oral medication or insulin). Only by doing so, you can better manage your daily blood glucose levels, and keep your diabetes under tight control.

GLUCOMETER FOR HOME USE: CONTOUR NEXT METER [7]

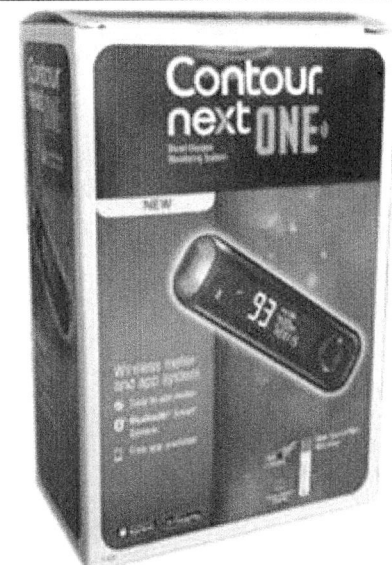	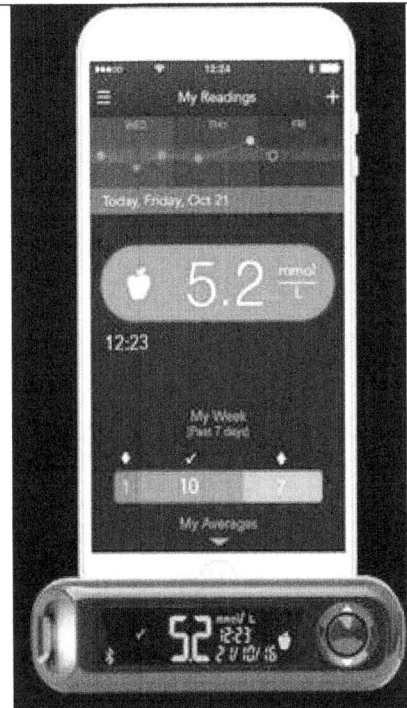
Traditional Blood Glucometer. [Also called patient's glucose meter] A simple and inexpensive glucometer for home use that suits everybody to do self-blood glucose monitoring every day. It comes with finger-stick test strips and lancets.	**Up-to-Date Glucometer** Meter can be hooked up to your smartphone.
Figure 2.5 Contour Next One Meter. Courtesy of Ascensia Diabetes Care Canada Inc.	Figure 2.6 Contour Nexe One Meter. Courtesy of Ascensia Diabetes Care Canada Inc.

You can better manage your diabetes by hooking up this up-to-date glucometer to your smartphone, and keep a record of all your blood glucose results and understand how your activities impact them, and take action in order to keep your diabetes under tight control. Contour next one meter would take the hassle out of your diabetes management, and help you understand your diabetes control. If you purchase this meter, the manufacturer (Bayer or Ascensia Diabetes Care Canada Inc.) trains you over the phone on how to use it, and even send you a meter for free. Or, a local pharmacist could teach you how to use the meter correctly.

IMPORTANT NOTE: Whenever you go to do your diabetes panel blood tests in a laboratory (once every 3 months), take this meter with you to the laboratory, and get it tested, and make sure it is working perfectly. Compare your meter reading with the result obtained from the lab analysis.

CONTINUOUS GLUCOSE MONITORING DEVICES

1. Dexcom G6 Continuous Glucose Monitoring (CGM) System [8] (Noninvasive Glucose Monitoring System Without Finget Prick)

Continuous Glucose Monitoring (CGM) is a noninvasive method to track glucose levels throughout the day and night without finger-poking. A CGM system takes glucose measurements at regular intervals, up to 24 hours a day, and translate the readings into dynamic data, providing complete information on how your blood glucose levels are fluctuating throughout the day. A CGM can also contribute to improve diabetes management by helping to minimize the guesswork that comes with making treatment decisions based solely on a number from a blood glucose meter reading. Studies have shown that Dexcom CGM systems help lower hemoglobin A1c level to normal with minimal efforts, and reduce hypoglycemia, whether users are on oral medications, insulin injections or pump therapy.

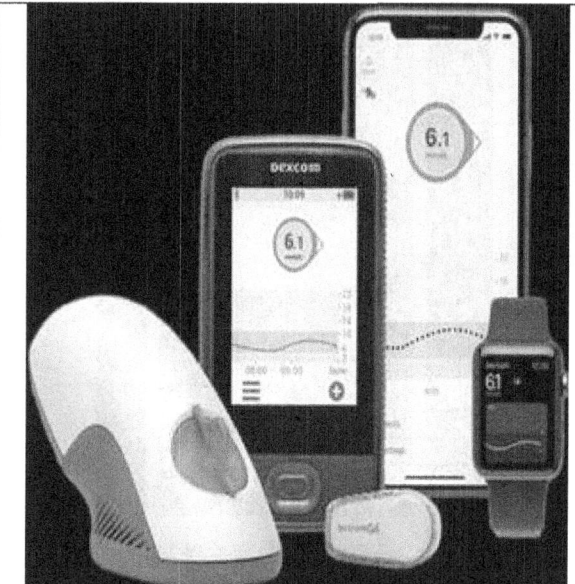

Figure 2.8 Dexcom G6 CGS System. Courtesy of Dexcom Inc.

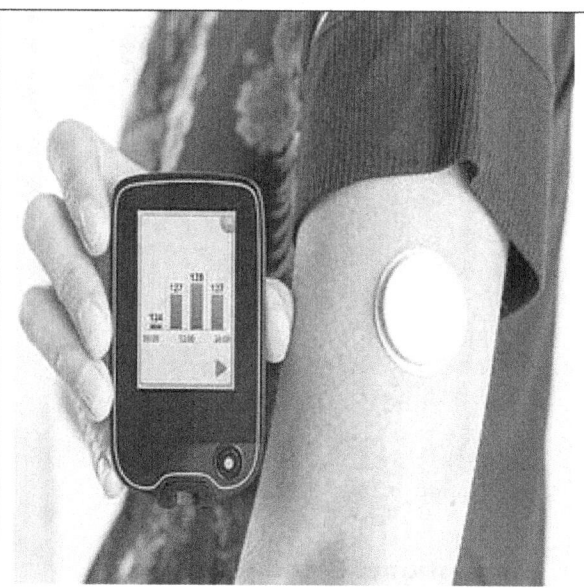

Figure 2.7 FreeStyle Livre 14-Day System. Courtesy of Abbott Laboratories

2. FreeStyle Livre Continuous Device With A 14-Day Sensor [9]

A small sensor automatically measures and continuously stores glucose readings day and night. The sensor lasts up to 14 days. Every 14 day, a new sensor has to be used. Glucose readings are recorded with a painless, one-second scan even through clothing. With every scan you get your current glucose reading, the last 8 hours of glucose data and an arrow showing the direction your glucose is heading. The FreeStyle Libre system is designed to be water-resistant and can be worn while bathing, showering, swimming or exercising.

Advantages: With a continuous device, you can very easily control diabetes, and achieve normal hemoglobin A1c. By watching the glucose level throughout the day, and by injecting the appropriate amount of insulin whenever the glucose level is too high, you can slash glucose spikes, and achieve normal average blood glucose level on a daily basis.

Disadvantages: The sensors are very expensive, and the people with low income cannot afford to purchase them. The people with low income can still use the traditional glucometer, and can still control diabetes by monitoring frequently, recording and analysing the blood glucose data manually without purchasing those expensive devices.

ROUTINE TESTS FOR DIABETICS [1]

If a person is diagnosed with diabetes (type 1, type 2, or gestational diabetes), he/she must perform the following tests in a laboratory, with the physician's requisition in your area, once every 3 months or at least every 6 months, depending on the severity of the situation.

1. Fasting Glucose and Hemoglobin A1c: Fasting glucose and Hemoglobin A1c tests must be performed once every 3 months in order to know if your diabetes is controlled or not.
2. Hematology Panel: A series of tests to understand the blood and diseases in blood.

3. Cholesterols Panel Tests: Total cholesterol, LDL cholesterol, HDL Cholesterol, Chol-HDL Ratio, Non HDL-Cholesterol, Triglycerides level. All these tests should be normal.
4. Thyroid Tests: TSH, T3 & T4.

5. Kidney Test & Urine Test: Estimated GFR (Glomerular Filtration Rate) test tells how quickly the kidneys are clearing waste from your body. Creatinine also suggests a kidney problem. Microalbumin (protein) level in urine tells if the kidneys are damaged.
6. Liver Test: ALT (Alanine Aminotrabsferase), AST (Aspartate Aminotransferase), LD (Lactate dehydrogenase). These tests pre-indicate the liver disease or liver damage. During the trial of a new cholesterol-lowering drug (mostly statin drugs), these tests must be performed and results verified once every month until the drug suits your body.

7. Blood Pressure: Between 60 and 65% of diabetic people suffer from high blood pressure. Frequent self-blood pressure testing is necessary at least once every week.

8. Vision Test: An Optometrist or Eye Specialist performs eye examination to check the development of cataracts, and to make sure that the Retina is normal and that there is no diabetes-related vision impairment.

9. Foot Care: The Family Physician, Endocrinologist or Neurologist organizes a physical examination to check the numbness in feet and knees, and to make sure that the feet are not affected by neuropathy or peripheral neuropathy.

10. Skin Care: An Endocrinologist or Dermatologist could identify skin problems related to diabetes and recommend a treatment.

11. SCAN Test: A Neurologist organizes a scan test, along with a physical examination, to make sure that neuropathy (nerve damage) is not caused by diabetes.

12. PSA Test: A Urologist examines the prostate gland and orders a urine test and PSA test to make sure the prostate is normal. Bladder tests are performed if you have urinary problems.

13. Stress Test: A Cardiologist usually organizes a stress test: Running on the treadmill to evaluate the heart condition. One can self-organize this treadmill test by going to a gym.

14. Doppler Test: A Vascular Specialist organizes a Doppler test to confirm the leg arteries are not narrowed (claudication) due to diabetes, which causes pain in lower legs while walking. This test confirms whether or not narrowing of leg arteries occured.

15. Dental Care: A General Dentist or a Specialist in periodontics could check for gum disease developed due to diabetes. Regular dental hygiene cleaning or deep gum cleaning once every 3 months is recommended for diabetic people.

HOW IS THE BLOOD GLUCOSE LEVEL EXPRESSED FOR DIABETES? [1]

In USA, Asia, and in most of the other countries around the world, blood glucose level is expressed in mg/dL. In Canada, UK, Australia, New Zealand, South Africa, and in some other countries, blood glucose level is expressed in mmol/L. If a diabetic person travels to other countries, and gets the blood test done, he/she should be educated enough to understand the test result in both units of measurement. The conversion factor is 18.

If you simply multiply the value in mmol/L by 18, you get the value in mg/dL.
If you simply divide the value in mg/dL by 18, you get the value in mmol/L.

For example, blood glucose level in Canada = 7 mmol/L
The same blood glucose level in USA = (7 mmol/L)(18) = 126 mg/dL

For example, the blood glucose level in USA = 160 mg/dL
The same blood glucose level in Canada or UK = (160 mg/dL)/(18) = 8.9 mmol/L

So a diabetic person must be familiar with both units, and should know how to convert the blood test result from one unit to the other.

WHY IS THE GLUCOSE CONVERSION FACTOR 18? [1]

Notation: dL = deciliter (1 liter = 10 deciliters); mg = milligram (1 gram = 1000 milligrams); mmol = millimole (1 mole = 1000 millimoles); L = liter

Sample Calculation
Molecular Formula of Glucose is: $C_6 H_{12} O_6$

Molecular Weight = (6)(12) + (12)(1) + (6)(16) = 72 + 12 + 96 = 180 mg/mmol (approximately)

Molecular Weight of Glucose = 180.16 mg/mmol (precisely)

Suppose the blood glucose level is reported by a laboratory in Canada as 5.8 mmol/L. Convert the blood glucose level value to mg/dL as expressed in the USA.

To convert from mmol/L to mg/L, multiply by molecular weight.
To convert from mg/L to mg/dL, divide by 10 (1 liter is equal to 10 deciliters).

    5.8 mmol/L = (5.8 mmol/L) (180.16 mg/mmol) / (10 dL/L)
               = 104.49 mg/dL

Or, simply multiply by the conversion factor 18.
    5.8 mmol/L = (5.8 mmol/L) (18) (mg/dL) / (mmol/L) = 104.49 mg/dL

Conversion Factor = (180.16 mg/mmol) / (10 dL/L)
                          = 18 (mg/dL) / (mmol/L)

To convert mmol/L of glucose to mg/dL, simply multiply by 18.
To convert mg/dL of glucose to mmol/L, simply divide by 18.

NORMAL BLOOD GLUCOSE LEVELS [1, 11, 12]

A diabetic person should be familiar with the normal blood glucose levels, and should make sure from a fingerstick blood test that the glucose levels are within the normal range. Frequent self-blood glucose tests are necessary to make sure that the diabetes is under tight control.

Table 2.2 Normal blood glucose levels of healthy (non-diabetic) people.

Normal Blood Glucose Levels of Healthy Non-Diabetic People [Courtesy of Joslin Diabetes Center, Adapted from One Touch Meter Manual]		
	Glucose (mmol/L)	Glucose (mg/dL)
Between 2 am and 4 am	> 3.9	> 70
Before breakfast (fasting)	3.9 to 5.8	70 to 105
Before lunch or before dinner	3.9 to 6.1	70 to 110
1 hour after meals	< 8.9	< 160
2 hours after meals	< 6.7	< 120

Table 2.3 Normal level of hemoglobin A1c.

Hemoglobin A1c	Normal Range
(i) Healthy Non-Diabetic People	4.5% - 6.2%
(ii) Diabetic People	< 7%

An Example of Diabetes Control

A highly self-disciplined diabetic person committed to control his/her diabetes and decided to achieve normal hemoglobin A1c in 3 to 6 months. He/she started self-monitoring 7 times a day (4 fasting glucose levels and 3 after-meal glucose levels) as shown in the table below:

Table 2.4

Time	7:15	9:00	12:00	14:00	18:45	19:45	22:00	**Average**
Glucose (mmol/L)	5.8	8.9	6.5	8.5	5.9	13.8	7.7	8.2
Glucose (mg/dL)	104.4	160.2	117	153	106.2	248.4	138.6	146.8

He/she calculated the daily average glucose level as 8.2 mmol/L or 146.8 mg/dL.

He/she took action to lower after meal glucose levels by means of the healthy diet, daily exercise, oral medication or insulin shots. After 3 to 6 months of consistent and serious efforts, the after-meal blood glucose levels, and daily average glucose level, dropped significantly as shown in the table below:

Table 2.5

Time	7:15	9:00	12:00	14:00	18:45	19:45	22:00	**Average**
Glucose (mmol/L)	5.2	7.5	6.5	7.2	5.9	10.5	6.7	7.1
Glucose (mg/dL)	93.6	135	117	129.6	106.2	189	120.6	127.3

HERE IS THE SECRET: If the daily average blood glucose level of a diabetic person is close to 7 mmol/L or 126 mg/dL for 90 consecutive days, the hemoglobin A1c will automatically normal. You can find this secret in the Hemoglobin A1c Chart.

REFERENCES

1. Permanent Diabetes Control (Book), Subtitle: The Complete Guide to Living Like A Normal Person Forever, Authored by Rao Konduru, MS, PhD, Reviewed and Endorsed by Dr. Marshal Dahl, MD, PhD., Endocrinologist, Faculty of Medicine, University of British Columbia, Vancouver, British Columbia, Canada, First Published in 2003.
www.mydiabetescontrol.com

2. Diabetes: Facts, Statistics, and You by Healthline.
https://www.healthline.com/health/diabetes/facts-statistics-infographic#1

3. YouTube Video, Title: What is Pancreas?, Published by Rahul Azad, Aug 24, 2009
https://www.youtube.com/watch?v=1l2GTGEwZOY&feature=youtu.be

4. YouTube Video, Title: How the Body Works: The Pancreas, Published by Daniel Izzo, Aug 3, 2017
https://www.youtube.com/watch?v=j5WF8wUFNkI&feature=youtu.be

5. Diabetes Overview by Mayo Clinic Staff, 2019.
https://www.mayoclinic.org/diseases-conditions/diabetes/symptoms-causes/syc-20371444

6. Type 2 Diabetes by Mayo Clinic, 2019.
https://www.mayoclinic.org/diseases-conditions/type-2-diabetes/diagnosis-treatment/drc-20351199

7. Contour Next One Meter Hooked Up to Smartphone by Ascensia Diabetes Care Canada Inc.
https://www.contournextone.ca/

8. What is Continuous Glucose Monitoring (CGM)? by Dexcom.com.
https://www.dexcom.com/en-CA/what-cgm

9. FreeStyle Libre Continuous Glucose Monitor Without A Finger Prick by abbott Laboratories.
https://www.freestyle.abbott/ca/en/products/libre.html

10. The Secret to Controlling Type 2 Diabetes, Subtitle: Addendum to Permanent Diabetes Control, Authored by Rao Konduru, Published in 2019, ISBN # 9780973112054, Available on Amazon.com, www.mydiabetescontrol.com

11. Krall, L.P, MD, and Beaser, R.S, MD, Joslin Diabetes Manual, Philadelphia, Lea and Febiger, Pages 3-6, 135, 138, 1989.

12. Glucose Ranges in People Without Diabetes, Lifescan's One Touch Profile Blood Glucose Monitoring Manual, Table on Page 51, Lifescan, Printed in USA, 1996.

CHAPTER 3 DIABETES CONTROL

TABLE OF CONTENTS

	Page
CHAPTER 3: DIABETES CONTROL	33
[A Very Important Chapter if You Are Diabetic]	
DIABETES CONTROL BASICS	35
▸ Introduction to Diabetes Control	35
▸ Control Your Diabetes in 90 Days: Why 90 Days?	36
▸ Hemoglobin A1c & Hemoglobin A1c Chart Explained	36
▸ Normal Blood Glucose Levels & Normal Hemoglobin A1c Levels	38
▸ The Secret to Controlling Diabetes Successfully	38
▸ Example 1 & Example 2 to Understand the Secret	39
▸ Can the Hemoglobin A1c Be Determined At Home?	39
▸ How to Calculate Daily Average Blood Glucose Level?	41
▸ WHO CAN USE ORAL MEDICATIONS & WHO CAN USE INSULIN SHOTS?	43
HOW TO CONTROL DIABETES	44
METHOD 1: Type 2 Diabetes Control	45
With **Healthy Diet & Exercise (No Medication)**	
▸ Dietary Guidelines	45
▸ Physical Activity Stimulates the Insulin Production from Pancreas	46
▸ EXAMPLE 1: How to Control Type 2 Diabetes	46
With Healthy Diet, Daily Exercise & Self-Discipline!	
▸ Disadvantages of Method 1	48
METHOD 2: Type 2 Diabetes Control	49
With **Healthy Diet, Oral Medication & Exercise**	
▸ Dietary Guidelines & Oral Medication	49
▸ Physical Activity Stimulates the Insulin Production from Pancreas	50
▸ EXAMPLE 2: How to Control Type 2 Diabetes	50
With Healthy Diet, Oral Medication, Daily Exercise & Self-Discipline!	
▸ Disadvantages of Method 2	52
METHOD 3: Type 2 Or Type 1 Diabetes Control	55
With **Healthy Diet, Insulin Shots & Exercise**	
▸ Introduction	55
▸ Uncontrolled Diabetes Is Dangerous	55
▸ Insulin Is The Best Medication For Diabetes	55
▸ Important Note On Insulin	56
▸ Dietary Guidelines & Rapid-Acting Insulin	56

	Page
▶ Physical Activity Stimulates the Insulin Production from Pancreas	57
▶ Physical Activity Also Stimulates the Artificial Insulin Injected	58
▶ How Much Artificial Insulin Is to be Injected?	58
▶ Physical Activity Cuts Insulin Dose In Half	58
▶ Hands On Training Course In A Diabetes Clinic	59
▶ FIVE IMPORTANT PRECAUTIONS	59
▶ How to Achieve Normal A1c With Insulin Shots & Exercise?	62
• How to Enjoy High Carbohydrate Meals & Slash After-Meal Glucose Spikes?	62
• FIVE EXAMPLES DISCUSSED WITH DAILY DIABETES CONTROL ROUTINE	62
• Example 3, Example 4, Example 5, Example 6, Example 7	62
▶ Advantages of Method 3	73
▶ Disadvantages of Method 3	73
▶ Why Should the Insulin Dose Be Optimized?	74
▶ How to Optimize Insulin Dose by Trial & Error?	74
▶ Trial & Error Procedure: Simplified Approach	75
• For A Small Meal, Mid-Sized Meal & Large Meal	
▶ Trial & Error Procedure: Sophisticated Approach	77
▶ Trial & Error Procedure: Diabetes Control (Flow Sheet)	78
▶ Dr. RK's Diabetes Has Been Controlled Permanently	79
▶ Official Blood Test Results of the Controlled Diabetes	79
▶ CLOSING REMARKS	81
▶ WHAT IS PERMANENT DIABETES CONTROL?	81
◉ REFERENCES	81
◉ About the Author	83

DIABETES CONTROL BASICS

INTRODUCTION TO DIABETES CONTROL [1]

When the pancreas of the human body produces little or no insulin, diabetes develops. Due to this insulin deficiency, the human body becomes unable to supply and control insulin flow in the bloodstream, thereby allowing elevated blood glucose levels. An artificially injected insulin dose is therefore essential to combat insulin deficiency. In order to properly optimize and utilize the artificially injected insulin action, diabetes should be controlled by simultaneously adjusting the food intake, daily exercise, the dosage of either oral medication or insulin. For a given major meal, the dosages of either oral medication or insulin dose and exercise should be simultaneously adjusted, which is a complex task to be practiced by a regular diabetic patient. Diabetes control can be simplified by keeping exercise as a constant factor, for a given major meal of known calories and/or carbohydrates, and by adjusting the dosage of either oral medication or insulin in an attempt to control mostly the after-meal glucose levels. The insulin dose can be approximately determined and cut in half or even less than half through by introducing after-meal exercise, self-monitoring after-meal glucose levels, and by analysing the blood glucose data. Attaining such an extensive monitoring and researching experience is not impossible, but it takes diligence, self-discipline, determination, commitment and a strong desire to live longer and healthy.

Diabetes control is considered to be a matter of controlling the following three parameters:

a. Fasting Glucose Level Before All Meals
b. After-meal Glucose Level (Within and After 2 Hours of the Meal)
c. Hemoglobin A1c (Monitored Once Every 3 Months)

An extensive study of after-meal meal glucose levels is essential in the beginning, for a period of 3 to 6 months, in order to research and understand the body's response with a variety of heavy meals against insulin dose and exercise. This research is unavoidably required to control diabetes that has long been forgotten and was left uncontrolled. After the hemoglobin A1c has been successfully brought close to normal value for the first time, the earned research experience helps guide the individual to further control diabetes without finger-poking as frequently. The individual who earns extensive research experience in the beginning for 3 to 6 months will be rewarded for the rest of his/her life.

A diabetic person should have a thorough knowledge about the normal blood glucose levels, and should be able to recognize how high or how low the glucose level is at any particular time. The blood glucose level of a non-diabetic person after 2 hours of a heavy meal consumption drops to normal range. For a diabetic person, it is indeed possible to lower the blood glucose level close to normal value within 2 hours of meal consumption through injecting appropriate insulin dose and introducing an after-meal exercise for one hour.

Normal Range of Blood Glucose Levels

Between 4 mmol/L and 7 mmol/L (In Canada, UK, Australia, New Zealand, South Africa).
Between 72 mg/dL and 126 mg/dL (In USA, Asia, and many other countries).

CONTROL YOUR DIABETES IN 90 DAYS: Why 90 Days? [1]

Most people with diabetes focus their attention on fasting glucose levels in order to control diabetes, rather than on lowering after-meal glucose levels. If your blood glucose level from a fingerstick blood test early in the morning is normal, it doesn't mean your diabetes is controlled. Hemoglobin A1c is a parameter that directly reveals the degree of "diabetes control" during the preceding 90 days. **Red blood cells live in the bloodstream for 90 days.** Every 90 days, new red blood cells are born. Hemoglobin is a protein molecule that ia present in red blood cells and carries and supplies oxygen from the lungs to the trillions of body's cells wherever it is needed. Hemoglobin also carries glucose along with it, because glucose can stick to all kinds of proteins in your body. While the blood circulates, depending on how high or how low the blood glucose level is, a certain amount of glucose is attached to the hemoglobin molecules to form glycated hemoglobin. Different doctors or scientists call it with different names: glycated A1c, hemoglobin A1c (HbA1c), or simply A1c. Therefore, by measuring the hemoglobin A1c level in a laboratory from the patient's blood sample, it is possible to know the average blood glucose level and the degree to which it has been controlled over the preceding 90 days. Which obviously means that it takes at least 90 days to see any improvement in the hemoglobin A1c level from a laboratory blood test.

HEMOGLOBIN A1c EXPLAINED [1]

Human blood, referred to as the river of life, is pumped from the heart through a network of large and small blood vessels. If all blood vessels and capillaries were joined together in one line, they would stretch to 300 million feet. Blood runs at different speeds depending on how fast the heart beats. A normal adult possesses about 5 to 6 liters of blood that is approximately 7 to 8 % of body weight. Blood is a liquid stored in the heart, blood vessels and in the sinusoids of the bone marrow, liver and spleen. About 55% of blood is plasma, a clear yellowish liquid. The other 45% of blood is made of red blood cells, white blood cells and platelets. Platelets coagulate when the skin is cut and form a clot to stop bleeding. Plasma is watery, consisting of 93% water and 7% solid proteins the majority of which is albumin. Bone marrow is a soft tissue located in bones that produces red blood cells, platelets and white blood cells. Plasma transports red blood cells, white blood cells and platelets through the blood vessels. Plasma delivers nutrients to trillions of cells and also picks up waste including carbon dioxide from the cells.

The blood carries oxygen from the lungs to all the body's cells where it is burned. But the oxygen could react quickly in blood and burn prematurely before it reaches the body's cells. This premature burning is prevented by a protein molecule. The blood in the human body contains about 30 trillion red blood cells, and each red blood cell has about 270 million protein molecules. Each protein molecule represents a ring composed of carbon, nitrogen and hydrogen atoms. The ring floats in the bloodstream and a cluster of 4 iron atoms that sit in the center of each ring protects a pair of oxygen atoms from premature burning. **This incredibly designed protein molecule is called "hemoglobin".**

Hemoglobin carries oxygen with it and drops it off whenever and wherever oxygen is needed in order to promote all sorts of chemical reactions that occur every instant in the body. Red blood cells live in the bloodstream for 60 to 90 days. Every 90 days, new red blood cells are generated in the bloodstream. While the blood circulates, glucose is attached to hemoglobin depending on how much glucose is present in the bloodstream. This attachment takes place in different ways and all the hemoglobin that is attached to glucose in the red blood cells is called "glycohemoglobin," roughly 6% of the hemoglobin in the blood. [2] The hemoglobin that is attached or bound to glucose is also called glycosylated hemoglobin. The more glucose is in the blood, the more glycohemoglobins or glycosylated hemoglobins form. Glycohemoglobin remains in the blood for 60 to 90 days. Glycohemoglobin is divided into 3 types such as A1a, A1b and A1c. Two-thirds of this glycohemogobin is called hemoglobin A1c, and one-third is made up of A1a and A1b. Hemoglobin A1c that is present in the red blood cells has special characteristics and is easily identifiable by laboratory techniques. This suggests that hemoglobin A1c reflects the total amount of glucose attached to it in red blood cells over the preceding 90 days. The measurement of hemoglobin A1c therefore indicates how high the average blood glucose level has been and how good/poor the blood glucose control has been over the preceding 90 days.

Analytical methods have been developed to readily test the diabetic person's blood and report the results of hemoglobin A1c test in "gm of A1c per gm of total hemoglobin" or in percentage (%). Medical scientists developed a correlation between hemoglobin A1c levels and the corresponding average blood glucose levels as shown in the table below. They found that lowering blood glucose level by 30 mg/dL (1.67 mmol/L) would lower hemoglobin A1c by approximately 1%, and decrease the diabetes risk probability by up to 25%.

For non-diabetic people, the normal level of hemoglobin A1c is between 4% and 6%. For diabetic people, a value less than 7% is considered "normal." Between 7% and 8% is considered fair, but not normal (you should try to lower it to 7). The following table or conversion chart shows the relationship between hemoglobin A1c and the average blood glucose level over the preceding 90 days.

HEMOGLOBIN A1c CHART [1]
[A Very Important Table to Keep in Mind if You Are Diabetic]

Table 3.1 Hemoglobin A1c Chart (Hemoglobin A1c Versus Average Blood Glucose).

HbA1c	Average Blood Glucose Level in 90 Days		
[%]	(mg/dL)	(mmol/L)	
4.0	60	3.3	It is Too Low, Try to Keep It Higher!
5.0	90	5.0	Perfectly Normal, Extremely Difficult to Achieve!
6.0	120	6.7	Normal, Very Good Control, Congrats!
6.2	126	7.0	Normal, Very Good Control (Reference Line)!
7.0	150	8.3	Fair or Moderately Good Control, Keep It Steady!
8.0	180	10.0	Too High, Take Action to Lower Immediately!
9.0	210	11.7	Poor Control, Take Action to Lower Immediately!
10.0	240	13.3	Poor Control, Take Action to Lower Immediately!
11.0	270	15.0	Very Poor Control, Take Action Immediately!
12.0	300	16.7	Very Poor Control, Take Action Immediately!
13.0	330	18.3	Very Poor Control, It Is Dangerous To Live Like That!
14.0	360	20.0	Very Poor Control, It Is Dangerous To Live Like That!
Courtesy of www.Bayer.com			

From this hemoglobin A1c chart, if you know the value of hemoglobin A1c from a laboratory blood test, you can determine the average blood glucose level in 90 days. Or, if you know the average blood glucose level in 90 days, you can determine the hemoglobin A1c level.

NORMAL BLOOD GLUCOSE LEVELS AND NORMAL A1c LEVELS [1, 3, 4]

Table 3.2 Normal blood glucose levels of healthy (non-diabetic) people.

Normal Blood Glucose Levels of Healthy Non-Diabetic People [Courtesy of Joslin Diabetes Center, Adapted from One Touch Meter Manual]		
	Glucose (mmol/L)	Glucose (mg/dL)
Between 2 am and 4 am	> 3.9	> 70
Before breakfast (fasting)	3.9 to 5.8	70 to 105
Before lunch or before dinner	3.9 to 6.1	70 to 110
1 hour after meals	< 8.9	< 160
2 hours after meals	< 6.7	< 120

Table 3.3 Normal level of hemoglobin A1c.

Hemoglobin A1c	Normal Range
(i) Healthy Non-Diabetic People	4.5% - 6.2%
(ii) Diabetic People	< 7%

The Secret to Controlling Diabetes Successfully [1]

Most diabetics don't know how to control diabetes, and live with uncontrolled diabetes, with elevated A1c level, for decades. Even the doctors and specialists are not equipped with the appropriate knowledge and training tools to transmit the real concept on controlling diabetes to the minds of their patients, except leaving their patients in a dilemma of uncontrolled diabetes. Read this section carefully and grasp the concept. If you understand this "secret", your diabetes control would be more rewarding than ever before, and this "secret" could save your life if you are seriously diabetic!

The secret lies in understanding the hemoglobin A1c Chart (Table 1.1) conceptually! Think like a mathematician by looking at the hemoglobin A1c chart "Average Blood Glucose Level Versus A1c", and try to understand how the chart was developed.

HERE IS THE SECRET: <u>If you can maintain your daily average blood glucose level at or below 7 mmol/L or 126 mg/dL every day for 90 consecutive days, your hemoglobin A1c would automatically be normal. You can find this secret in the Hemoglobin A1c Chart.</u>

Think about this concept over and over again, and program your mind to manage your daily average blood glucose level at or below 7 mmol/L or 126 mg/dL every day for 90 consecutive days, and then take the laboratory blood test. You will be surprised to learn that your hemoglobin A1c result is normal (close to 7% or 0.07).

Most people live with uncontrolled diabetes just because they were never taught this secret. Whenever your glucose level jumps above and beyond 7 mmol/L or 126 mg/dL, you need to compensate that excess by lowering it to below 7 mmol/L or 126 mg/dL, and by staying close to the lowest possible level so that the average glucose level would always be 7 mmol/L or 126 mg/dL.

EXAMPLE-I: For example, your after-meal glucose level rose to 10 mmol/L or 180 mg/dL and stayed there for 2 hours. Immediately after 2 hours, if you can lower that spike to 5 mmol/L or 90 mg/dL, and keep it lowered for another 3 hours, your average glucose level during the preceding 5 hours would be precisely 7 mmol/L or 126 mg/dL. If your average blood glucose level is 7 mmol/L or 126 mg/dL, your hemoglobin A1c would automatically be normal. You can understand this from basic arithmetics by simply calculating the average of 5 numbers (the total of 5 numbers divided by 5). This is a very simple example. If you can understand this simple example and solve this simple problem, you will be able solve much complex problem, by calculating average glucose level for all 24 hours. You don't need to calculate the average for all 24 hours, but just grasp the concept through your imagination.

EXAMPLE-II: For example, your after-meal glucose level rose to 10 mmol/L or 180 mg/dL and stayed there for 4 hours. Immediately after 4 hours, if you can lower that spike to 5 mmol/L or 90 mg/dL, and keep it lowered for another 6 hours, your average glucose level during the preceding 10 hours would be precisely 7 mmol/L or 126 mg/dL. your average blood glucose level is 7 mmol/L or 126 mg/dL, your hemoglobin A1c would automatically be normal. This is a very simple example. If you can understand this simple example and solve this simple problem, you will be able solve much complex problem, by calculating average glucose level for all 24 hours. You don't need to calculate the average for all 24 hours, but just grasp the concept through your imagination.

Bottom Line

Whenever the glucose level spikes above and beyond 7 mmol/L or 126 mg/dL, you should immediately lower that spike to 5 mmol/L or 90 mg/dL, and keep it lowered by staying close to lowest possible level so that the average glucose level would always be 7 mmol/L or 126 mg/dL. In other words, you need to compensate any excess glucose level in intervals of time throughout the day by lowering your glucose level to lowest possible value. It doesn't matter whether you are type 1 diabetic or type 2 diabetic, if you could master this concept, and could maintain you daily average at 7 mmol/L or 126 mg/dL for 90 consecutive days, your A1c would automatically be normal (< 7% or < 0.07). Your hemoglobin A1c is normal means your diabetes is tightly controlled.

Can The Hemoglobin A1c be Determined At Home? [1]
If You Understand This Example, Then You Understand A1c Chart!

It may sound unbelievable, but yes, hemoglobin A1c can be manually determined at home, without going to a laboratory for a blood test, up to a certain degree of accuracy using your fingerstick blood glucose meter. This kind of self-monitoring would help you control your diabetes on your own at home without anybody's help. You don't need to go to your doctor, get a requisition for blood test, and go to a laboratory to have the blood test done. You can approximately determine your hemoglobin A1c at home if you are knowledgeable, and eager to do it.

The following experiment will show you how to do it at home using your glucometer.
A diabetic person recorded his/her blood glucose levels (4 fasting glucose levels and 4 after-meal glucose levels) in a typical day as shown below using the glucometer at home:
Table 3.4

Time	7:15	9:00	12:00	14:00	18:45	19:45	22:00	23:00	Average
Glucose (mmol/L)	5.8	8.9	6.5	8.5	5.9	15.8	12.7	7.7	9.0
Glucose (mg/dL)	104.4	160.2	117	153	106.2	248.4	174.6	138.6	150.3

He/she then calculated the average glucose level as 9.0 mmol/L or 150.3 mg/dL.

IMPORTANT NOTE: By exercising high self-discipline and high willpower, he/she thus monitored blood glucose levels every day continuously, at least 6 to 8 times a day, without any interruption for 90 consecutive days, and calculated the average blood glucose value in 90 days as 9.2 mmol/L or 165.6 mg/dL. From the aforementioned A1c Chart (shown above in Table 5.1), he/she determined hemoglobin A1c value as approximately 7.5% or 0.075.

Average glucose level in 90 days = 9.2 mmol/L or 165.6 mg/dL
Hemoglobin A1c from the "A1c Chart" = 7.5% = 0.075

The more finger-stick blood glucose data a person collects, the more accurate the value of hemoglobin A1c would be. If you monitor 10 times a day (5 fasting glucose levels and 5 after-meal glucose levels for 90 consecutive days), your self-monitored hemoglobin A1c value would be more accurate (but it is still an approximate value, and not an exact value which is obtained from a laboratory blood test). If you can monitor every hour (24 times a day) for 90 consecutive days, and calculate the average blood glucose level, then your A1c would be reasonably accurate.

IMPORTANT NOTE (CAUTION): However, please be noted that the hemoglobin A1c test should be done in a laboratory once every 3 months to make certain that your diabetes is precisely controlled. The above-mentioned calculations would help you manage your diabetes tentatively and to lower your A1c to normal but do not provide you with accurate A1c value. You cannot always trust your glucometer at home and suppose that it is working perfectly. Your meter might be broken, you probably didn't even notice, and your meter could be producing erroneous results. If that happens, you will end up determining a wrong result of A1c. You cannot simply rely on the A1c value determined at home all the time. So it is very important that you need to find out your hemoglobin A1c value from a laboratory test once every 3 months and compare it with your self-monitored value every now and then. Also get your meter tested and make sure it is working perfectly whenever you go to a laboratory for your diabetes panel blood test.

HOW IS THE BLOOD GLUCOSE LEVEL EXPRESSED FOR DIABETES? [1]

In USA, Asia, and in most of the other countries around the world, blood glucose level is expressed in mg/dL. In Canada, UK, Australia, New Zealand, South Africa, and in some other countries, blood glucose level is expressed in mmol/L. If a diabetic person travels to other countries, and gets the blood test done, he/she should be educated enough to understand the test result in both units of measurement. The conversion factor is 18.

If you simply multiply the value in mmol/L by 18, you get the value in mg/dL.
If you simply divide the value in mg/dL by 18, you get the value in mmol/L.

For example, blood glucose level in Canada = 7 mmol/L
The same blood glucose level in USA = (7 mmol/L)(18) = 126 mg/dL

For example, the blood glucose level in USA = 160 mg/dL
The same blood glucose level in Canada or UK = (160 mg/dL)/(18) = 8.9 mmol/L

So a diabetic person must be familiar with both units, and should know how to convert the blood test result from one unit to the other.

HOW TO CALCULATE DALILY AVARAGE BLOOD GLUCOSE LEVEL? [2]
(THESE BASIC ARITHMETICS COULD SAVE YOUR LIFE!)

Now we will calculate the average glucose levels as shown below:

EXAMPLE-I: Calculate the average of 2 glucose levels
(1 fasting glucose level and 1 after-meal glucose level).

For example, fasting glucose level = 4 mmol/L
For example, after-meal glucose level = 10 mmol/L

$$\text{Average} = \frac{4 + 10}{2} = 7 \text{ mmol/L}$$

For example, fasting glucose level = 72 mg/dL
For example, after-meal glucose level = 180 mg/dL

$$\text{Average} = \frac{72 + 180}{2} = 126 \text{ mg/dL}$$

From the Hemoglobin A1c Chart, A1c = < 7% (which is normal).

If you know the average blood glucose level for 90 consecutive days, you can find out A1c from the A1c chart. The more times you monitor throughout the day, the more accurate your A1c would be. If your daily average is close to 7 mmol/L or 126 mg/dL for 90 days, your A1c will be normal.

EXAMPLE-II: Calculate the average of 4 glucose levels
(2 fasting glucose levels and 2 after-meal glucose levels).

For example, 2 fasting glucose levels are = 4 & 5 mmol/L
For example, 2 after-meal glucose levels are = 10 & 12 mmol/L

$$\text{Average} = \frac{4 + 10 + 5 + 12}{4} = 7.75 \text{ mmol/L}$$

For example, fasting glucose levels = 72 & 90 mg/dL
For example, after-meal glucose levels = 180 & 216 mg/dL

$$\text{Average} = \frac{72 + 180 + 90 + 216}{4} = 139.5 \text{ mg/L}$$

From the Hemoglobin A1c Chart, A1c = < 7% (which is normal).

If you know the average blood glucose level for 90 consecutive days, you can find out A1c from the A1c chart. The more times you monitor throughout the day, the more accurate your A1c would be. If your daily average is close to 7 mmol/L or 126 mg/dL for 90 days, your A1c will be normal.

EXAMPLE-III: Calculate the average of 6 glucose levels (3 fasting glucose levels and 3 after-meal glucose levels).

For example, 3 fasting glucose levels are = 4, 5 & 6 mmol/L
For example, 3 after-meal glucose levels are = 10, 12 & 15 mmol/L

$$\text{Average} = \frac{4 + 10 + 5 + 12 + 6 + 15}{6} = 8.7 \text{ mmol/L}$$

For example, 3 fasting glucose levels = 72, 90 & 108 mg/dL.
For example, 3 after-meal glucose levels = 180, 216 & 270 mg/dL

$$\text{Average} = \frac{72 + 180 + 90 + 216 + 108 + 270}{6} = 156 \text{ mg/L}$$

From the Hemoglobin A1c Chart, A1c = > 7% (which is not normal, take action to lower!).

If you know the average blood glucose level for 90 consecutive days, you can find out A1c from the A1c chart. The more times you monitor throughout the day, the more accurate your A1c would be. If your daily average is close to 7 mmol/L or 126 mg/dL for 90 days, your A1c will be normal.

Similarly you can calculate the average glucose level by monitoring 10 times a day, and determine haemoglobin A1c value from the A1c chart. The more times you monitor, the more accurate your A1c would be. If you monitor every hour (24 times a day) for 90 consecutive days, you haemoglobin A1c value would be reasonably accurate.

IMPORTANT NOTE: You can do this more accurately, and find out your hemoglobin A1c at home by using a continuous glucose monitoring device such as Dexcom System or FreeStyle Livre 14-Day System.

WHO CAN USE ORAL MEDICATIONS & WHO CAN USE INSULIN SHOTS?
[1, 2, 3]

The International Diabetes Federation (IDF) reported in 2017 that there are approximately 425 million adults worldwide (ranging 20-79 years of age) living with diabetes. About 5 to 10% of these people suffer from type 1 diabetes, and the remaining 90 to 95% suffer from to type 2 diabetes. [3]

Type 1 Diabetes: Type 1 diabetes mellitus or insulin-dependent diabetes mellitus or adult diabetes, also called juvenile diabetes, is developed when the pancreas produces little or no insulin because the beta cells of the pancreas may have been totally damaged or destroyed. Type 1 diabetes is developed mostly in infants, children and young adults under the age 30 years. Insulin shots are certainly required to treat type 1 diabetes. As explained above, in order to optimize the insulin dose and insulin action, type 1 diabetics also need to exercise after every major meal consumption in order to slash the after-meal spikes and to tightly control diabetes.

Type 2 Diabetes: Nearly 40% of the adults in USA alone suffer from pre-diabetes or borderline diabetes, and at least some of them would soon be diagnosed with type 2 diabetes. The people with type 2 diabetes around the world can be categorized into 3 groups based on the severity of the disease: (i) mild, (ii) moderate and (iii) severe.

- For those people with prediabetes or borderline diabetes, or mild type 2 diabetes, diabetes can be controlled without any oral medication or insulin, but with healthy lifestyle (dietary changes) and regular exercise or physical activity. However high self-discipline is required to maintain healthy lifestyle.

- For some people with moderate type 2 diabetes, diabetes can be controlled with healthy lifestyle (dietary changes), and oral medication (s) along with regular exercise or physical activity. However high self-discipline is required to maintain healthy lifestyle.

- For those people with severe type 2 diabetes, and for some people with moderate type 2 diabetes, oral medications do not work effectively, and it would be difficult to achieve normal hemoglobin A1c. And so this group of diabetic people are advised to switch to insulin shots (both long-acting insulin and rapid-acting) along with after-meal exercise. Those diabetics who use insulin shots need after-meal exercise because insulin dose needs to be optimized. Injecting too much insulin without exercise has adverse side effects, and therefore insulin dose should be cut in half by incorporating an appropriate after-meal exercise plan.

- Some diabetic people with expert knowledge go easy on the dietary guidelines and still manage to control diabetes with insulin shots, keep their A1c perfectly normal, and live like a normal person. These people with expert knowledge know how to inject the right amount of rapid-acting insulin, by trial and error and exercise, and lower after-meal blood glucose spike quickly to normal, and know how to achieve normal A1c.

▶ Insulin is the best medicine to treat diabetes, and insulin shots always work for any kind of diabetes (either type 1 diabetes or type 2 diabetes). That is why, many doctors recommend their patients to switch to insulin shots.

HOW TO CONTROL DIABETES

The next question pops up on your mind is how to lower that high after-meal blood glucose spike immediately to normal, and how to control diabetes?

There are three methods being discussed in this course with easy-to-understand examples: Method 1, Method 2 & Method 3. If you can lower your after-meal blood glucose spike to normal every day for 90 days in an attempt to lower your daily average blood glucose level close to 7 mmol/L or 126 mg/dL, your hemoglobin A1c comes down to normal (**THIS IS THE SECRET**). Dr. RK has been doing this successfully for the past 20 years.

Method 1: Type 2 Diabetes Control
HEALTHY DIET & EXERCISE WITHOUT ANY MEDICATION

Method 2: Type 2 Diabetes Control
HEALTHY DIET ALONG WITH ORAL MEDICATION & EXERCISE

Method 3: Type 2 Diabetes Control | Type 1 Diabetes Control
HEALTHY DIET ALONG WITH INSULIN SHOTS & EXERCISE

WHY ARE AFTER-MEAL BLOOD GLUCOSE LEVELS NOT TOO HIGH? AN IMPORTANT CLARIFICATION

By examining the self-blood glucose monitoring results in Method 1, Method 2, Method 3, a reader might wonder and raise a question such as "why are the after-meal blood glucose levels not significantly high enough in the collected glucose data?". Most of the data showed in these examples have after meal-glucose levels under 13 mmol/L or 234 mg/dL.
To understand this, please refer to Method 3 where "Ketones Formation" and "Ketoacidosis" are explained. A diabetic person should be cautious beforehand and should not exercise when the after-meal glucose levels are higher than 13 mmol/L or 234 mg/dL, unless the exercise suits his/her body without forming ketones. A diabetic person should inject the correct amount of insulin just before consuming a major meal to lower his/her blood glucose level close to 13 mmol/L or 234 mg/dL, and then exercise in order to lower his/her after-meal blood glucose level to perfectly normal (5 mmol/L or 90 md/dL). That is why in all the self-blood glucose monitoring data, you will find the after-meal blood glucose levels below 13 mmol/L or 234 mg/dL.

Method 1: Type 2 Diabetes Control
WITH HEALTHY DIET & EXERCISE (NO MEDICATION)

DIETARY GUIDELINES
After-meal spike of the blood glucose level can be avoided by consuming a low-carbohydrate meal without medication:

- A low-carbohydrate diet with lean meat (oven-baked skinless chicken, skinless turkey or fish), all kinds of vegetables, leafy greens, legumes, fruits (limited quantity only), low-fat milk or skim milk, and nut and seeds (limited quantity) is completely safe and healthy for a diabetic person. Every person, whether diabetic or non-diabetic, should eagerly try to eat a variety of vegetables, leafy greens and fruits available in the market by changing them every day, and by covering all of them every week so that the body would get all kinds of vitamins, minerals and fiber.
- A whole foods meal, without any processed or refined items in it, along with egg whites best suits a diabetic person. Egg whites is one 100% protein and one 100% safe, and so it can be used to adjust the daily protein requirement in order to balance any meal.
- White rice spikes blood glucose level immediately after consumption, and therefore a diabetic person (who is not on insulin) should never eat white rice. Brown rice or wild rice is okay, but it still needs control.
- Salt consumption and oil consumption should be minimized in order to lose weight and keep the blood pressure under control.
- A diabetic person should lose excess weight in order to control his/her diabetes. Weight loss could result in the reversal of type 2 diabetes, and keeps the blood pressure and cholesterols under control.
- A low-carbohydrate diet or no-carbohydrate diet with excessive amount of red meat, processed meat, or breaded and deep-fried meats for a diabetic person is unsafe, unhealthy, and even dangerous, and therefore should be avoided.
- Hamburgers, cheeseburgers, deep-fried potatoes (so called fries), all kinds of processed and refined products of any kind, all kinds of bakery items, all kinds of ready-to-eat meals, all kinds of breads, anything made by adding starchy white flour or all-purpose white flour, all kinds of soups and soup mixes, all kinds of chips and snacks being sold in supermarkets, grocery stores and gas stations could unwillingly and unnoticeably make a diabetic person overweight or obese and could clog and damage arteries, and therefore should be avoided.
- Always read the label whenever you purchase any food item, focus your attention on whole foods (natural foods). Make sure the food is not altered, processed or refined, and make sure that it does not contain any additives, preservatives, artificial colors and flavors except the food itself in its natural form.
- Alcohol abuse increases the lipids in the blood, which is a type of fat that can harden arteries, increasing bad cholesterol (LDL cholesterol) and arterial plaque in the heart's blood vessels and arteries. Eventually the arteries could be clogged, resulting in heart attack or heart failure. Therefore a diabetic person should avoid regular alcohol drinking.
- **Smoking poses** greater risk for people with diabetes. Just like high blood glucose levels, the poisonous chemicals in cigarette smoke attack blood vessels, contributes to hardening of the arteries (or what is known as atherosclerosis) which impairs the blood's ability to carry oxygen to the trillions of the body's cells. Eventually the arteries could be clogged, causing heart attack or heart failure. Therefore, a diabetic person should quit smoking immediately or as soon as possible.

▶ No medication is necessary if your diabetes is under control with diet and exercise.

PHYSICAL ACTIVITY STIMULATES THE INSULIN PRODUCTION FROM PANCREAS
Physical Activity (Any Kind of Exercise) Boosts Insulin Production from Pancreas

● The function of the islets of Langerhans is to produce two important hormones called insulin and glucagon (long chains of glucose). Beta cells of pancreas produce insulin and alpha cells of pancreas produce glucagon. The amazing counter-action between beta cells and alpha cells situated in the islets of Langerhans is responsible to maintain normal blood glucose levels. Physical activity has a significant positive effect on insulin sensitivity. Any type of physical activity stimulates beta cells in order to release more insulin, and has the potential to make your body's insulin work better by flowing smoothly throughout the blood vessels.

● Diabetes Care (a monthly peer-reviewed medical journal of American Diabetes Association) published the following information: In a randomized study on type 2 diabetes, researchers asked 1,152 Mexican Americans about their physical activity, and took blood samples to analyze their beta cell function of pancreases, and levels of glucose and insulin. They found that people who said they exercised had better beta cell function, independent of weight, diet, and body fat. The researchers concluded that the physical activity (daily exercise) may boost beta cells function of pancreas, releases more insulin into the bloodstream, thereby lowering blood glucose levels.

EXAMPLE: 1 How to Control Type 2 Diabetes With Dietary Guidelines
Mike was diagnosed with type 2 diabetes 5 years ago. But he has been living without diabetes care. He never tried to understand what diabetes is and never read a book about it. Even though his doctor warned him numerous times and insisted him to control diabetes, he has neglected all about his diabetes, and kept himself busy with his work, and has been eating greasy foods in all kinds of restaurants. Recently he had a minor heart attack and hospitalized for a few days. His doctors performed an angioplasty and told him that a bypass surgery is unnecessary at that time, and released him from the hospital.

After he came home from the hospital, he went to library and read as many diabetes books as possible. He also purchased several diabetes books online and read them all with curiosity. He most recently purchased "Permanent Diabetes Control", read it cover to cover, understood all the contents, and was indeed inspired to control his diabetes for the rest of his life. Now he has a clear concept on "how to control diabetes". He has also seen several diabetes nurses and endocrinologists, got answers to his questions, and also attended a diabetes course in his community diabetes center. He collected all the information, and equipped himself with all the tools necessary to control his diabetes. In other words, Mike awakened the giant within him, and committed to control his diabetes, starting today.

By consuming the same kind of meals (breakfast, lunch & dinner) he has been consuming during the past 5 years in a typical day, he monitored his blood glucose levels (4 fasting glucose levels and 4 after-meal glucose levels) using his self-monitoring glucose meter, and recorded as follows (just to do some research and to see what was going wrong):

Table 3.5

Time	7:15	9:00	12:00	14:00	18:45	19:45	22:00	23:00	Average	A1c
Glucose (mmol/L)	5.8	15.9	7.5	22.8	6.9	20.5	18.5	8.1	13.3	10%
Glucose (mg/dL)	104.4	286.2	135	410.4	124.2	369	333	145.8	238.5	10%

He then calculated the daily average blood glucose level as 13.3 mmol/L or 238.6 mg/dL. By using the A1c Chart (show above), he determined the hemoglobin A1c level as approximately 10%.

MIKE'S DIETARY CHANGES & EXERCISE PROGRAM

Mike committed to make dietary changes, and to exercise high self-discipline and high willpower. He immediately stopped eating out in the restaurants, and started cooking and eating at home. His new diet is shown below:

Breakfast: Puffed wheat cereals, low-fat milk (or soy milk) and a banana.
Lunch: Oven-baked chicken breast, legumes, salad made from leafy greens & tomatoes. He walked 30 minutes after lunch.
Dinner: Oven-baked fish, brown rice (limited quantity), steamed vegetables & an apple. He walked another 30 minutes after dinner.
Snacks: Limited quantities of cottage cheese (dry curd), salad, Kamut puffs, cashews, nuts & seeds (limited quantity), etc.
Water: He started drinking 8 to 16 cups of purified water. He also learned how to remineralize purified water.

As a result of the dietary changes and exercise, he lost weight, and his body mass index dropped to normal in a few months, and he did not have major after-meal blood glucose spikes anymore. Within a few days, his blood glucose levels in general dropped significantly. He continued to live like that for 90 days. His daily blood glucose monitoring data in a typical day are shown below:

Table 3.6

Time	7:15	9:00	12:00	14:00	18:45	19:45	22:00	23:00	Average	A1c
Glucose (mmol/L)	5.2	10.8	6.4	10.9	6.9	13.5	7.3	7.2	8.5	7.2%
Glucose (mg/dL)	93.6	194.4	115.2	196.2	124.2	243	131.4	129.6	153.5	7.2%

After 90 days, from the hemoglobin A1c chart, he determined the value of hemoglobin A1c as approximately 7.2%.
After 6 months, from the hemoglobin A1c chart, he determined the value of hemoglobin A1c as approximately 7.0%.
After 1 year, from this hemoglobin A1c chart, he determined the value of hemoglobin A1c as approximately 6.7%.

Once every 3 months, he took diabetes panel blood test in a laboratory, and his hemoglobin A1c was found to be normal (< 7%).

Mike is happier than ever. His diabetes is reasonably controlled, and will remain controlled for the rest of his life as long as:
- He self-monitors and records his blood glucose levels every day, calculates daily average, and tries to keep his daily average close to 7 mmol/L or 126 mg/dL every single day,
- He eats healthy meals at home by following the dietary guidelines, and avoids eating junk foods (processed foods & refined foods) in restaurants,
- He walks or exercises in a gym every day after a major meal consumption,
- He exercises high self-discipline and high willpower to maintain the normal A1c level (<7%).

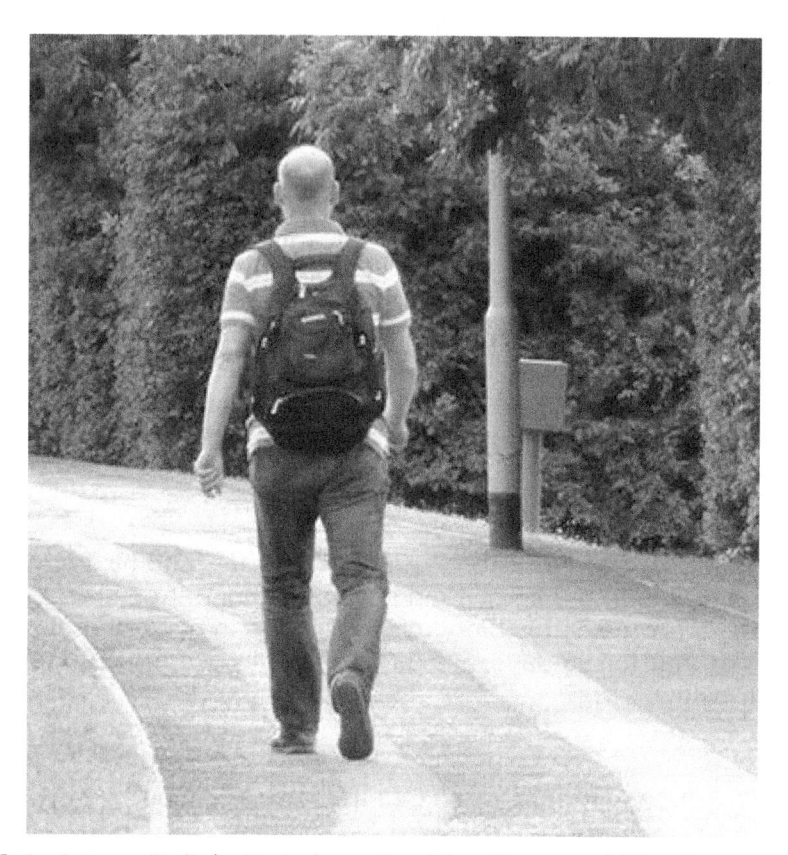

Figure 3.1 A type 2 diabetic is lowering his after-meal blood glucose levels with the aid of exercise (walking on the road).

DISADVANTAGES OF METHOD 1 (WITHOUT MEDICATION)
- It works for some people only (mostly for pre-diabetics). It doesn't work for most people with diabetes. You need to try it out looking for successful results.
- Even if it works, after some time it may not work, and the person may eventually need an oral medication or insulin.
- It is extremely difficult to maintain high self-discipline and high will power, and so most people cannot maintain normal A1c level all the time. People eat out every now and then, tempt to eat snacks and other unsafe foods, and diabetes could easily go out of control.

Method 2: Type 2 Diabetes Control
WITH HEALTHY DIET, ORAL MEDICATION & EXERCISE

DIETARY GUIDELINES
After-meal spike of the blood glucose level can be avoided by consuming a low-carbohydrate meal along with medication:
● A low-carbohydrate diet with lean meat (oven-baked skinless chicken, skinless turkey or fish), all kings of vegetables, leafy greens, legumes, fruits (limited quantity only), low-fat milk or skim milk, and nut and seeds (limited quantity) is completely safe and healthy for a diabetic person. Every person, whether diabetic or non-diabetic, should eagerly try to eat a variety of vegetables, leafy greens and fruits available in the market by changing them every day, and by covering all of them every week so that the body would get all kinds of vitamins, minerals and fiber.
● A whole foods meal, without any processed or refined items in it, along with egg whites best suits a diabetic person. Egg whites is one 100% protein and one 100% safe, and so it can be used to adjust the daily protein requirement in order to balance any meal.
● White rice spikes blood glucose level immediately after consumption, and therefore a diabetic person (who is not on insulin) should never eat white rice. Brown rice or wild rice is okay, but it still needs control.
● Salt consumption and oil consumption should be minimized in order to lose weight and keep the blood pressure under control.
● A diabetic person should lose excess weight in order to control his/her diabetes. Weight loss could result in the reversal of type 2 diabetes, and keeps the blood pressure and cholesterols under control.
● A low-carbohydrate diet or no-carbohydrate diet with excessive amount of red meat, processed meat, or breaded and deep-fried meats for a diabetic person is unsafe, unhealthy, and even dangerous, and therefore should be avoided.
● Hamburgers, cheeseburgers, deep-fried potatoes (so called fries), all kinds of processed and refined products of any kind, all kinds of bakery items, all kinds of ready-to-eat meals, all kinds of breads, anything made by adding starchy white flour or all-purpose white flour, all kinds of soups and soup mixes, all kinds of chips and snacks being sold in supermarkets, grocery stores and gas stations could unwillingly and unnoticeably make a diabetic person overweight or obese and could clog and damage arteries, and therefore should be avoided.
● Always read the label whenever you purchase any food item, focus your attention on whole foods (natural foods). Make sure the food is not altered, processed or refined, and make sure that it does not contain any additives, preservatives, artificial colors and flavors except the food itself in its natural form.
● Alcohol abuse increases the lipids in the blood, which is a type of fat that can harden arteries, increasing bad cholesterol (LDL cholesterol) and arterial plaque in the heart's blood vessels and arteries. Eventually the arteries could be clogged, resulting in heart attack or heart failure. Therefore a diabetic person should avoid regular alcohol drinking.
● Smoking poses greater risk for people with diabetes. Just like high blood glucose levels, the poisonous chemicals in cigarette smoke attack blood vessels, contributes to hardening of the arteries (or what is known as atherosclerosis) which impairs the blood's ability to carry oxygen to the trillions of the body's cells. Eventually the arteries could be clogged, causing heart attack or heart failure. Therefore, a diabetic person should quit smoking immediately or as soon as possible.
▶ **An oral medication** similar to "Metformin (Glucophage® XR)" has to be taken with the evening meal or according to the dosage instructions provided by the

manufacturer. Sometimes, your doctor may also prescribe you a second oral medication such as Invokamet. Some doctors also prescribe insulin sensitizers such as Actos, which helps your body to use the insulin from the pancreas effectively and at the same time decreases the glucose released by the liver. However there are many oral medications for type 2 diabetes.

PHYSICAL ACTIVITY STIMULATES THE INSULIN PRODUCTION FROM PANCREAS
Physical Activity (Any Kind of Exercise) Boosts Insulin Production from Pancreas

- The function of the islets of Langerhans is to produce two important hormones called insulin and glucagon (long chains of glucose). Beta cells of pancreas produce insulin and alpha cells of pancreas produce glucagon. The amazing counter-action between beta cells and alpha cells situated in the islets of Langerhans is responsible to maintain normal blood glucose levels. Physical activity has a significant positive effect on insulin sensitivity. Any type of physical activity stimulates beta cells in order to release more insulin, and has the potential to make your body's insulin work better by flowing smoothly throughout the blood vessels.

- Diabetes Care (a monthly peer-reviewed medical journal of American Diabetes Association) published the following information: In a randomized study on type 2 diabetes, researchers asked 1,152 Mexican Americans about their physical activity, and took blood samples to analyze their beta cell function of pancreases, and levels of glucose and insulin. They found that people who said they exercised had better beta cell function, independent of weight, diet, and body fat. The researchers concluded that the physical activity (daily exercise) may boost beta cells function of pancreas, releases more insulin into the bloodstream, thereby lowering blood glucose levels.

EXAMPLE: 2 How to Control Type 2 Diabetes With Dietary Guidelines and Oral Medication

Both parents of Maria were diagnosed with type 2 diabetes when they were in their sixties. According to the Centers for Disease Control and Prevention (CDC), type 2 diabetes accounts for about 90 to 95 percent of all diagnosed cases of diabetes in adults, and type 1 diabetes accounts for the remaining 5 to 10 percent. Diabetes is known to be hereditary. The influence of family history on whether a person develops diabetes is better established with type 2 than it is with type 1. When Maria was 55 years old, she suffered from frequent urination problem, and was hospitalized for a couple of days. An endocrinologist (diabetes specialist), in the hospital, ordered a diabetes panel blood test, and diagnosed her with type 2 diabetes. The hospital staff asked Maria many questions concerning her family history and diabetes sufferers in her family, and concluded that the heredity was the reason why Maria's was diagnosed with with type 2 diabetes. The laboratory blood test showed the following results:

Her fasting glucose level (from the laboratory blood test) was 9.5 mmol/L or 171 mg/dL
Her hemoglobin A1c (from the laboratory blood test) was 11.3%

On the same day, the nurses researched about her eating habits and the rise and fall of her daily blood glucose levels during 24 hours period. They gave Maria exactly the same kind of meals she has been consuming at her home in a typical day, and monitored her blood glucose levels (4 fasting glucose levels and 4 after-meal glucose levels). Maria's blood glucose levels in a typical day, when she was diagnosed with type 2 diabetes, are shown below:

Table 3.7

Time	6:00	9:00	12:00	14:00	18:45	19:45	22:00	23:00	Average	A1c
Glucose (mmol/L)	9.2	19.5	8.9	22.5	10.8	19.7	18.5	9.8	14.9	11.0%
Glucose (mg/dL)	165.6	351	160.2	405	194.4	354.6	333	176.4	267.5	11.0%

They calculated the average glucose level in a typical day as 14.9 mmol/L or 267.5 mg/dL.
They determined her hemoglobin A1c (from A1c Chart) as roughly 11%.
Maria is supposed to take action immediately and lower A1c.

The endocrinologist in the hospital prescribed her Metformin alone (Glucophage® XR), 500 mg once a day with evening meal.

Type 2 Diabetes Training Course

Maria was asked by her doctor to take a type 2 diabetes training course in the same hospital. A nurse taught her in a 2-day session all about the dietary changes, how to eat healthy, how to count calories, how to take oral medication, and how to exercise every day after a major meal consumption. Maria came home and started controlling her diabetes seriously. She purchased the finger-stick blood glucose monitor, strips and lancets. She purchased the medication Metformin alone (Glucophage® XR), 500 mg, enough for 3 months (to be re-filled once every 3 months).

Self-Monitoring Daily Blood Glucose Levels

She started monitoring her blood glucose levels 8 times a day (4 farting glucose levels & 4 after-meal glucose levels). She learned how to calculate the daily average glucose level. She also learned how to estimate her hemoglobin A1c level roughly using A1c Chart. She is also committed to take diabetes panel tests once every 3 months in a laboratory. She is also scheduled to see her endocrinologist (diabetes specialist) once every 3 months.

After 6 months of dieting and exercise along with oral medication, her blood glucose level data on a typical were recorded as follows:

Table 3.8

Time	6:00	9:00	12:00	14:00	18:45	19:45	22:00	23:00	Average	A1c
Glucose (mmol/L)	6.9	13.5	7.5	15.8	7.5	13.0	10.8	7.5	10.3	8.3%
Glucose (mg/dL)	124.2	243	135	284.4	135	234	194.4	135	185.6	8.3%

Maria calculated the average glucose level in a typical day as 10.3 mmol/L or 185.6 mg/dL.
Maria also determined her hemoglobin A1c (from A1c Chart) as roughly 8.3%.

Her fasting glucose level (from the laboratory blood test) was 6.5 mmol/L or 117 mg/dL
Her hemoglobin A1c (from the laboratory blood test) was 8.6%
Her hemoglobin A1c dropped from 11.3% to 8.6% in 6 months.
That was a great improvement, but it still need further control.
So her endocrinologist (diabetes specialist) increased the dosage of her medication to 1000 mg.
After 12 months (6 months after increasing the dosage of her medication to 1000 mg), and after making some more changes to her diet and exercise, her blood glucose level data on a typical were recorded as follows:

Table 3.9

Time	6:00	9:00	12:00	14:00	18:45	19:45	22:00	23:00	Average	A1c
Glucose (mmol/L)	5.3	10.2	7.5	10	5.8	9.7	7.5	6.0	7.8	6.8%
Glucose (mg/dL)	95.4	183.6	135	180	104.4	174.6	135	108	139.5	6.8%

Maria calculated the average glucose level in a typical day as 7.8 mmol/L or 139.5 mg/dL. Maria also determined her hemoglobin A1c (from A1c Chart) as roughly 6.8%.

Her fasting glucose level (from the laboratory blood test) was 4.9 mmol/L or 88 mg/dL
Her hemoglobin A1c (from the laboratory blood test) was 6.9%
Her hemoglobin A1c dropped from 11.3% to 6.9% in 12 months, which is considered normal for a diabetic person.

Once every 3 months, she took diabetes panel blood test in a laboratory, and her hemoglobin A1c was found to be normal (< 7%).

Maria is happier than ever. Her diabetes is reasonably controlled, and will remain controlled for the rest of her life as long as:
◦ She self-monitors and records her blood glucose levels every day, calculates daily average, and tries to keep her daily average close to 7 mmol/L or 126 mg/dL every single day.
◦ She eats healthy meals at home, and avoids eating junk foods (processed foods & refined foods) in restaurants,
◦ She takes her oral medication every day with her evening meal, and never forgets,
◦ She walks or exercises in a gym every day after a major meal consumption,
◦ She exercises high self-discipline and high willpower to maintain normal A1c level (<7%).

DISADVANTAGES OF METHOD 2 (WITH ORAL MEDICATION)
◦ It is extremely difficult to maintain high self-discipline and high will power. Most people cannot maintain normal A1c level all the time. They eat out every now and then, tempt to eat snacks and other unsafe foods, and so diabetes could easily go out of control.
◦ It works for some people and it doesn't work for other people with diabetes. You need to try it out looking for successful results.
◦ It takes long time to see successful results (where as with insulin shots, you can see immediate results with perfection).
◦ Even if it works, after some time it may not work, and the person may eventually need insulin.
◦ For most diabetics, it is not possible to accomplish perfect diabetes control with consistent hemoglobin A1c level.
◦ Pills don't work as effectively as insulin. Artificial insulin is the best medication for diabetes, as explained in Method 3.

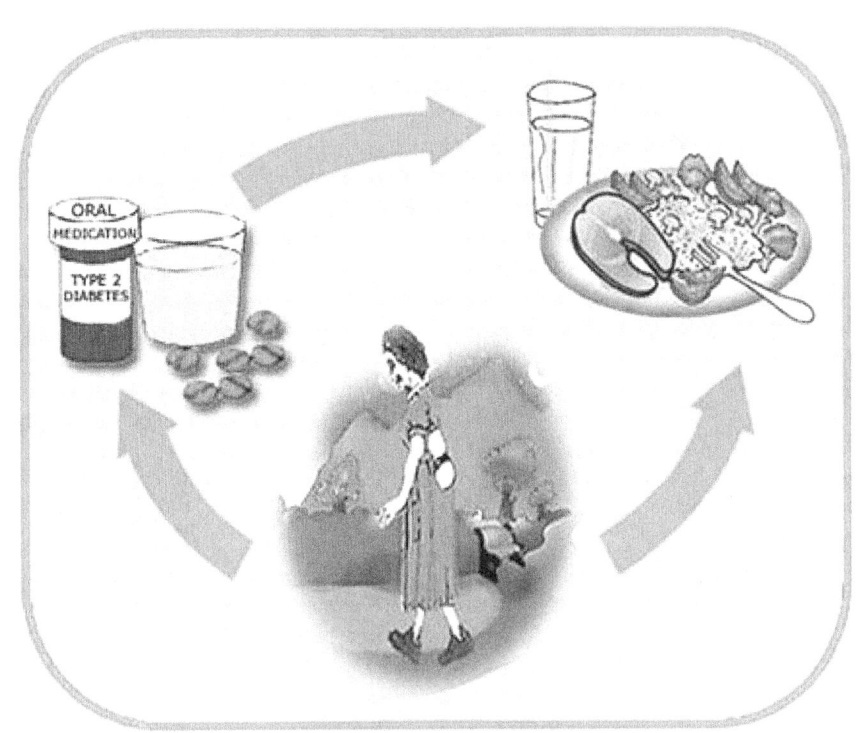

Figure 3.2 A type 2 diabetic is lowering her after-meal blood glucose level with the aid of oral medication and exercise (Walking on the Road).

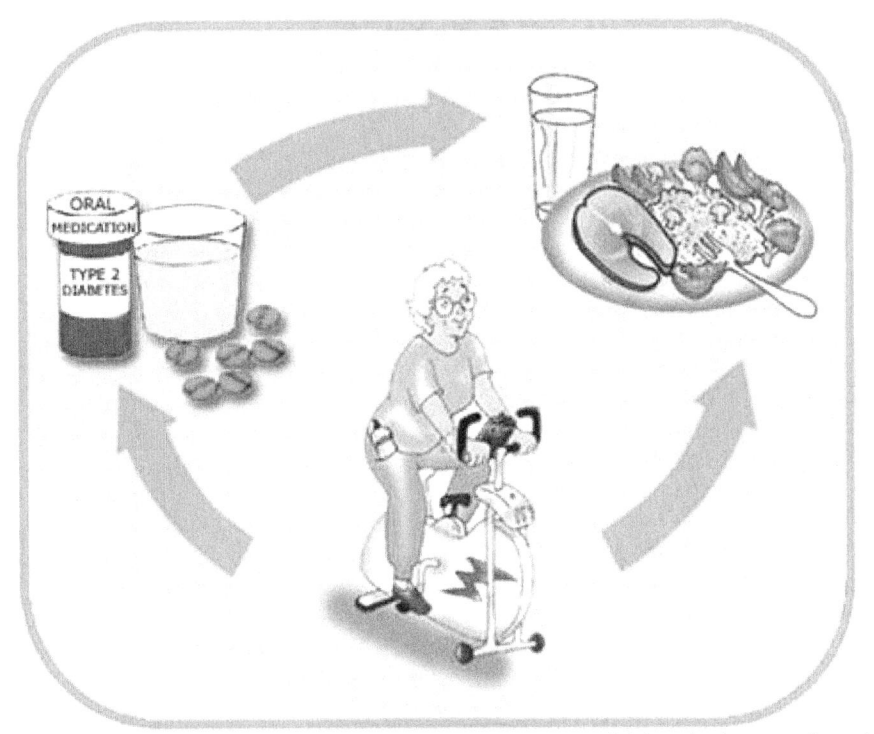

Figure 3.3 A type 2 diabetic is lowering her after-meal blood glucose level with the aid of oral medication and exercise (Biking in a Gym).

Method 3: Type 2 Diabetes Control
WITH HEALTHY DIET, INSULIN SHOTS & EXERCISE

INTRODUCTION: If the oral medication along with diet and exercise does not stabilize your blood glucose levels and if you are unable to maintain a consistently normal A1c (<7%), then you should switch to insulin injections, and your diabetes control would be more rewarding than ever. Pills don't work for many people. It is a slow process to see successful results of maintaining normal A1c. But insulin is guaranteed to work instantly. You can see results immediately within an hour in terms of lowering blood glucose levels. Even if you are type 2 diabetic, you can always switch to insulin shots any time without any fear or hesitation. Many type 2 diabetics around the world use insulin shots to control diabetes.

UNCONTROLLED DIABETES IS DANGEROUS
Don't simply rely on oral medications, waste year after year, and live with uncontrolled diabetes. Living with uncontrolled diabetes, and neglecting your health by inadequately managing your chronic diabetes means you are living with high glucose levels in the bloodstream, and high levels of hemoglobin A1c. At elevated blood glucose levels over a long time, the glucose sticks to the surface of the cells and it is then converted into a poison called "sorbitol", which damages the body's cells and blood vessels, leading to long-term side effects such as:

- High cholesterols (total cholesterol & LDL cholesterol) and high blood pressure,
- Heart attack, heart failure, coronary heart disease, stroke,
- Hardening of arteries or what is known as atherosclerosis,
- Peripheral artery disease (PAD), narrowing of arteries,
- Painful neuropathy (nerve damage and poor blood flow),
- Burning foot syndrome, numbness in feet and knees, intermittent claudication,
- Amputation (due to nerve damage in the feet),
- Kidney disease, kidney damage, loss of kidney,
- Erectile dysfunction (ED) and/or Impotence,
- Cataracts, blurred vision, retinopathy, blindness,
- Deafness (hearing impairment),
- Diseases of the small blood vessels in the eyes, kidneys, legs and nerves,
- Gum disease and bone loss (dental problems),
- Bladder and prostate problems,
- Skin diseases (bacterial and fungal infections),
- Dementia such as Alzheimer's disease,
- Depression develops over time if diabetes is left untreated,
- and many other strange problems and complications.

If your hemoglobin A1c is more than 7%, your diabetes in uncontrolled, so take action immediately! When after-meal blood glucose spike is too high after eating and remain elevated for more than two hours, this presents a significant mortality risk factor, and the person should switch to insulin shots.

INSULIN IS THE BEST MEDICATION FOR DIABETES
A rapid-acting insulin such as Humalog or Novolog/NovoRapid, if combined with exercise, would help lower the blood glucose spike immediately and is guaranteed to work instantly if you know exactly how many units you needed to inject.
▶ A highly knowledgeable diabetic person can very easily lower his/her huge blood glucose spike to perfectly normal within 30 minutes by injecting the right amount of insulin and by running on a treadmill.

You will not be able to lower a huge blood glucose spike with oral medications being prescribed. A rapid-acting inhaled insulin Afrezza is a new oral medication, but it is not yet widely known in all places (not available in Canada). Even if it is available, it cannot be divided into tiny portions. Whereas insulin can be injected in tiny doses as you like.

Even the biking or walking on the street, with insulin injected, would help lower the steep blood glucose spike. If you inject the right amount of insulin for a given meal you consumed, and run on a treadmill for 30 minutes, for example, your blood glucose spike drops immediately from a high-risk 20 mmol/L or 360 mg/dL to a stunning 5 mmol/L or 90 mg/dL. And then if you could keep this average glucose level at 7 mmol/L or 126 mg/dL for the rest of the day, your daily average would be perfectly normal. If you can keep up the daily average blood glucose level close to 7 mmol/L or 126 mg/dL for 90 consecutive days, your A1c will automatically be normal. You will become a master of diabetes control, your life will change, and you will be happier than ever.

IMPORTANT NOTE ON INSULIN
Rapid-acting insulin such as Humalog or Novolog alone doesn't work effectively. Rapid-acting insulin works only on the top of the long-acting insulin such as Humulin-N. Whenever you inject rapid-acting insulin such as Humalog, you should have long-acting insulin such as Humulin-N already injected into your body. Whenever you switch to insulin shots, you should always use both long-acting insulin (Humalog) and rapid-acting insulin (Humulin-N) together. You should master the concept of how insulin works, and how to inject. You should go to your community diabetes center, and take a "full course" on how to use insulin shots for diabetes. They will train you and teach you on how to calculate insulin doses and how to inject (it doesn't matter if you are type 1 diabetic or type 2 diabetic).

However, you need to research and find out which method (of the 3 methods discussed above) suits you the best, and stick to that treatment. Switching to insulin shots would be the best choice, it doesn't matter at all weather you are type 2 diabetic or type 1 diabetic. You can always switch from one method to the other.

DIETARY GUIDELINES & RAPID-ACTING INSULIN
After-meal spike of the blood glucose level can be avoided by consuming a low-carbohydrate meal along with insulin shots.
- A low-carbohydrate diet with lean meat (oven-baked skinless chicken, skinless turkey or fish), all kings of vegetables, leafy greens, legumes, fruits, low-fat milk or skim milk, and nut and seeds (limited quantity) is completely safe and healthy for a diabetic person. Every person, whether diabetic or non-diabetic, should eagerly try to eat a variety of vegetables, leafy greens and fruits available in the market by changing them every day, and by covering all of them every week so that the body would get all kinds of vitamins, minerals and fiber.
- A whole foods meal, without any processed or refined items in it, along with egg whites best suits a diabetic person. Egg whites is one 100% protein and one 100% safe, and so it can be used to adjust the daily protein requirement in order to balance any meal.
- White rice, brown rice, wild rice, or any other high-carbohydrate whole food meal can be consumed as long as the diabetic person knows how to inject the right amount of insulin and exercise thereafter, and lower your after-meal glucose spike to perfectly normal within 1 or 2 hours.
- Salt consumption and oil consumption should be minimized in order to lose weight and keep the blood pressure under control.

- A diabetic person should lose excess weight in order to control his/her diabetes. Weight loss could result in the reversal of type 2 diabetes, and keeps the blood pressure and cholesterols under control.
- A low-carbohydrate diet or no-carbohydrate diet with excessive amount of red meat, processed meat, or breaded and deep-fried meats for a diabetic person is unsafe, unhealthy, and even dangerous, and therefore should be avoided.
- Hamburgers, cheeseburgers, deep-fried potatoes (so called fries), all kinds of processed and refined products of any kind, all kinds of bakery items, all kinds of ready-to-eat meals, all kinds of breads, anything made by adding starchy white flour or all-purpose white flour, all kinds of soups and soup mixes, all kinds of chips and snacks being sold in supermarkets, grocery stores and gas stations could unwillingly and unnoticeably make a diabetic person overweight or obese and could clog and damage arteries, and therefore should be avoided.
- Always read the label whenever you purchase any food item, focus your attention on whole foods (natural foods). Make sure the food is not altered, processed or refined, and make sure that it does not contain any additives, preservatives, artificial colors and flavors except the food itself in its natural form.
- Alcohol abuse increases the lipids in the blood, which is a type of fat that can harden arteries, increasing bad cholesterol (LDL cholesterol) and arterial plaque in the heart's blood vessels and arteries. Eventually the arteries could be clogged, resulting in heart attack or heart failure. Therefore a diabetic person should avoid regular alcohol drinking.
- Smoking poses greater risk for people with diabetes. Just like high blood glucose levels, the poisonous chemicals in cigarette smoke attack blood vessels, contributes to hardening of the arteries (or what is known as atherosclerosis) which impairs the blood's ability to carry oxygen to the trillions of the body's cells. Eventually the arteries could be clogged, causing heart attack or heart failure. Therefore, a diabetic person should quit smoking immediately or as soon as possible.

▶ Rapid-acting insulin such as Humalog is to be injected just before or immediately after every meal consumption (breakfast, lunch, dinner, and all snacks). Long-acting insulin has to be injected once or twice a day. Rapid-acting insulin does not work effectively if there no long-acting insulin in your body.

If you master the concept of injecting rapid-acting insulin, you can go easy on the aforementioned dietary guidelines, and enjoy high carbohydrate meal once or twice a week. Some diabetic people with expert knowledge go easy on the aforementioned dietary guidelines and still manage to control diabetes with insulin shots, keep their A1c perfectly normal, and live like a normal person. You cannot do that with oral medications. So it is strongly advised to switch to insulin shots if you are type 2 diabetic.

PHYSICAL ACTIVITY STIMULATES THE INSULIN PRODUCTION FROM PANCREAS
Physical Activity (Any Kind of Exercise) Boosts Insulin Production from Pancreas
- The function of the islets of Langerhans is to produce two important hormones called insulin and glucagon (long chains of glucose). Beta cells of pancreas produce insulin and alpha cells of pancreas produce glucagon. The amazing counter-action between beta cells and alpha cells situated in the islets of Langerhans is responsible to maintain normal blood glucose levels. Physical activity has a significant positive effect on insulin sensitivity. Any type of physical activity stimulates beta cells in order to release more insulin, and has the potential to make your body's insulin work better by flowing smoothly throughout the blood vessels.

● Diabetes Care (a monthly peer-reviewed medical journal of American Diabetes Association) published the following information: In a randomized study on type 2 diabetes, researchers asked 1,152 Mexican Americans about their physical activity, and took blood samples to analyze their beta cell function of pancreases, and levels of glucose and insulin. They found that people who said they exercised had better beta cell function, independent of weight, diet, and body fat. The researchers concluded that the physical activity (daily exercise) may boost beta cells function of pancreas, releases more insulin into the bloodstream, thereby lowering blood glucose levels.

PHYSICAL ACTIVITY ALSO STIMULATES THE FLOW OF ARTIFICIAL INSULIN INJECTED

● Artificial insulin is synthesized in such a way that it works much more effectively and flows a lot more quickly throughout the blood vessels with physical activity (exercise). The amount of artificial insulin dosage must be minimized (optimized) because:

◆ Too much insulin lowers blood glucose level too fast, causing hypoglycemia (a disorder of low blood glucose levels).

◆ Too much insulin also constricts arteries, leading to heart attack and coronary heart disease.

◆ Too much insulin also stimulates the brain so that a person feels hungry and eats more and causes the liver to manufacture fat in the belly.

◆ Too little insulin on the other hand would not be enough to cover the entire meal and to maintain normal glucose levels.

◆ **An optimum insulin dose is therefore crucial**. After-meal exercise, either treadmill, biking or walking, should be introduced into the diabetes control plan in order to burn fat, lose calories and optimize both the insulin dose and insulin action. After-meal exercise minimizes the insulin dose and maximizes insulin action and prevents after-meal glucose levels from rising too high, thus keeping diabetes under tight control.

HOW MUCH ARTIFICIAL INSULIN IS TO BE INJECTED TO CONTROL DIABETES? GENERAL RULE

▶ The insulin manufacturing company Eli Lily recommended that in general 1 unit of rapid-acting Humalog is necessary for 8 grams of carbohydrate in your meal in order to lower after-meal glucose level to normal. This rule is being used in all the diabetes clinics around the world.

◆ If you consume 80 g of carbohydrate through your meals, you need to inject 10 units of Humalog insulin.

◆ If you consume 100 g of carbohydrate through your meals, you need to inject 12.5 units of Humalog insulin.

◆ If you consume 200 g of carbohydrate through your meals, you need to inject 25 units of Humalog insulin.

◆ And so on.

PHYSICAL ACTIVITY (EXERCISE) CUTS INSULIN DOSAGE REQUIREMENT IN HALF

If you consume 80 g of carbohydrate through your meals, and if you are not exercising and staying home, you need to inject 10 units of Humalog insulin to lower your after-meal glucose level to normal or close to normal.

If you consume 80 g of carbohydrate through your meals, and are planning to exercise (running on a treadmill or biking in a gym, or walking on the road or in the shopping mall), you need to inject only 5 units of Humalog insulin (insulin dose has to be cut in half). After 30 minutes of exercise, your blood glucose level drops to normal. Some people need to inject the remaining 5 units of Humalog (2nd shot) after completing the exercise in order to keep the after-meal glucose levels normal for a prolonged period of time. Some people don't need the second shot. You need to research on yourself, and find out the right rapid-acting insulin dose for any given meal.

HANDS ON TRAINING COURSE IN A DIABETES CLINIC IN YOUR AREA

If you are planning to switch to insulin shots, you should take a training course in a local diabetes clinic in your community or nearby hospital. The hands on training course is a diabetes clinic is usually organized by an endocrinologist (diabetes specialist), a nurses and a dietician, for a few days. They teach you:

a. How to inject insulin (both long-acting insulin and rapid-acting insulin) into the fatty tissue of your body,
b. How to find out the amount of carbohydrate in any meal,
c. How to count calories using measuring cups or by weighing foods with an electronic balance,
d. How to calculate the dosage of rapid-acting insulin for any meal, and
e. How to exercise to lower after-meal glucose levels to normal by running on a treadmill or by walking with rapid-acting insulin injected.

Once you have learned everything about diabetes control with insulin and exercise, you can go home and start controlling your diabetes with insulin shots. Your diabetes control would be more rewarding than ever (a lot better than the treatment with oral medications). You can achieve perfect diabetes control if you work hard.

FIVE IMPORTANT PRECAUTIONS
Every insulin-dependant diabetic should be aware of the following 5 precautions:

1. **HYPOGLYCEMIA (Low Blood Glucose Levels):** If you are going to try rapid-acting insulin shots with exercise (treadmill or other) in order to control your diabetes, in the beginning stages until you become accustomed to this treatment, you should monitor after every 15 minutes or as frequently as possible, and make sure your blood glucose level did not drastically drop to below normal 5 mmol/L or 90 mg/dL, and did not reach a condition called hypoglycemia (low blood glucose levels). If you inject too much insulin and run on a treadmill or walk, your blood glucose level may drop below normal, and you may be collapsed or knocked out due to hypoglycemia. Be aware and beware of this dangerous situation, and protect yourself by monitoring every 15 minutes or at least every 30 minutes. Always carry concentrated sugar solution or sugar jelly with you so that you swallow sugar and recover quickly from any such predicament. Chewing a candy sometimes helps raise blood glucose level.

2. **KETONES FORMATION:** If you exercise when your blood glucose level is above 14 mmol/L or 250 mg/dL, and if there is not enough insulin in your body because you are diabetic (either type 1 or type 2), your body becomes unable to use glucose as fuel and starts burning fat, releasing ketones into your body. Ketones (chemically known as ketone bodies) are byproducts of the breakdown of fatty acids. Glucose is the body's main source of energy. In order to transport glucose to trillions of body's cells, you need insulin. But when the body cannot use glucose for energy because of lack insulin, it burns fat instead, and uses as energy. When fats are broken down for energy, chemicals

called ketones appear in the blood and urine. When some obese people, who are seriously diabetic and whose blood glucose levels are too high after eating (above 14 mmol/L or 250 mg/dL), go on strenuous exercise, their bodies burn fat because of the lack of insulin in the body, and burning fat may lead to a serious condition called diabetic ketoacidosis (DKA), which requires immediate medical treatment.

The Symptoms of ketoacidosis (DKA) Are: nausea, feeling of illness, vomiting, abdominal pain, common cold or flu, tiredness all the time, thirsty or very dry mouth, flushed skin, difficulty breathing, confusion, and fruity breath. If you notice any of these symptoms when your blood glucose level is above 14 mmol/L or 250 mg/dL, and when exercising, you should immediately do a blood ketone test (you can also do urine ketone test, but it is not accurate), and find out if you have developed ketones formation in your body, and take action immediately. If ketones are present, you should stop exercising, and immediately inject a rapid-acting insulin such as Humalog to lower the blood glucose level to below 14 mmol/L or 250 mg/dL.

Some people do exercise with rapid-acting insulin injected when blood glucose level is above 14 mmol/L (or 250 mg/dL), and do not experience any formation of ketones or pertinent symptoms. Every person is different, and therefore you should research and be prepared to face such situation (how to avoid or handle the ketones formation).

♦ To avoid any such unsafe situation of ketones formation, you should inject rapid-acting insulin just before and during the high-carbohydrate meal consumption so that your after-meal glucose level will not be elevated above and beyond 14 mmol/L or 250 mg/dL. Then you can exercise without panicking about ketones formation.
♦ Or you should consume a well-planned healthy diet that will not raise your blood glucose level above 14 mmol/L or 250 mg/dL, and exercise thereafter without panicking about ketones formation.

3. **ARTIFICIAL INSULIN SENSITIVITY:** Artificial insulin sensitivity varies from person to person. Some people may need more units of insulin (both long-acting insulin and rapid-acting insulin), and some others may need less units insulin for the same amount of high-carbohydrate meal and for the same length of exercise to lower the after-meal glucose level to normal. Each person is different so he/she should research, and find out the appropriate insulin dose for a particular meal. By trial and error, and by monitoring every 15 minutes, you should be able to determine the right insulin dose for a particular high-carbohydrate meal, and stick to that insulin dose when repeating the same meal next day. As the experience builds up, you will be able to guess the insulin dose quickly for any given meal, and inject it to lower after-meal glucose level like an expert.

PLEASE NOTE: As the insulin manufacturing company Eli Lily suggested "1 unit of rapid-acting insulin Humalog is required for every 8 grams of carbohydrate being consumed", it may not be true for all people. One unit of Humalog per 8 grams of carbohydrate is a rough estimate to begin with. It could be a little more a little less depending on the body's ability to handle the artificial insulin. Some obese people may need more insulin to control after-meal glucose levels than the others. Every person has to research and find out, by trial and error, exactly how many units of rapid-acting insulin are to be injected for a particular meal. Rapid-acting insulin works on the top of long-acting insulin so you should not try using rapid acting insulin alone.

4. **ARTIFICIAL INSULIN RESISTANCE:** Artificial insulin resistance is very commonly encountered by the people with diabetes who inject rapid-acting insulin (Humalog) every day and exercise to lower after-meal glucose levels. Suddenly insulin stops working even if you double or triple the dosage (number of units of rapid-acting insulin) because the body developed insulin resistance. If that happens, the best natural remedy is to go on fasting for a couple of days to a week, and consume low-calorie and non-fat soups, organic apple cider vinegar with mother unfiltered and unpasteurized and lemon juice with cayenne pepper throughout the day, and you should lose weight at least a few pounds. After a few days to a week, you will notice yourself that the insulin resistance disappeared, and insulin starts working as usual.

5. **LIPOHYPERTROPHY (INSULIN SHOTS OVER TIME DEVELOP ABDOMINAL LUMPS):**

If you start using insulin shots, you better understand what "Lipohypertrophy" is. Lipohypertrophy is a medical term, meaning a lump under the skin, caused by the accumulation of extra fat at the site of many subcutaneous injections of insulin. It may be unsightly and mildly painful, and may interfere with insulin action. Insulin may not work as effectively as expected if you developed lipohypertrophy. It is a common complication caused due to carelessly managed injections on the abdominal. To avoid lipohypertrophy, never re-use the syringes (discard the syringe after every sigle use), and do not inject insulin repeatedly at the same site of your belly or any other body part. Keep rotating injection sites every day. Divide your abdominal into 4 quadrants. Inject on 1st quadrant during the first week, by leaving a half an inch between every two injection sites, and proceed to next quadrant during the next week, and so on. Many insulin-dependant diabetic people suffer from abdominal lumps because they were not properly trained when they started injecting insulin shots. So if you are new to insulin shots, you better be aware of this problem called "lipohypertrophy" beforehand.

If you have already developed lipohypertrophy, the following are the treatment methods:

(i) Massage the lumps with your hand regularly by applying baby oil (you will see improvement day by day). The lumps may not disappear completely, but you will see some improvement.
(ii) Seek laser treatment with a specialist (most likely a plastic surgeon could do it) if lumps are bothering you. If the lumps are not bothering, you can live with them.
(iii) Liposuction is also heard to be a quick and ideal treatment to remove a large abdominal lumps,
(iv) Ultrasound body fat reduction treatment is also being used by some doctors.
(v) Electricity therapy is also available to treat lipohypertrophy.

Longer Needles, Or Shorter Needles? [5]

In the past, diabetics have been using 12.7 mm needles to inject insulin. Most recently, research proved that a needle depth of 5 mm works fine for all people, including children. With shorter needles (4 to 5 mm), inject at a 90-degree angle with no pinching of the skin. If longer needles are used, pinch up the skin to avoid injecting into intramuscular tissue. Also, hold the needle in the skin for 5 to 10 seconds after you give the insulin (even longer with higher doses) so the medication doesn't leak from the site. For very lean people, pinching the skin and injecting at an angle are recommended even with shorter needles.

HOW TO ACHIEVE NORMAL A1c WITH INSULIN SHOTS & EXERCISE? FIVE EXAMPLES DISCUSSED WITH DAILY DABETES CONTROL ROUTINE

EXAMPLE: 3 How to Control Type 2 Diabetes With Insulin & Exercise
This Is The Most Important Example If You Want To Enjoy High-Carbohydrate Meals and Still Live With Normal A1c

INTRODUCTION: Adam was diagnosed with type 2 diabetes when he was 46 years old. Adam tried Method 1 (Dietary Guidelines Without Oral Medication) for a year. It did not work. Then he started using Method 2 (Dietary Guidelines Along With Oral Medication) for two more years. It did not work for him because he could not maintain high self-discipline and high will power, and has been cheating on his diet, and eating in restaurants every now and then. His hemoglobin A1c has been very high, and was unable to lower it significantly. He changed doctors and visited several endocrinologists, and also tried several kinds of oral medications in all possible dosages. Those oral medications did not work. He wasted altogether 4 to 5 years, trying oral medications, without any success. He could not lower his hemoglobin A1c to close to 7%. His hemoglobin A1c has always been above and beyond 9.5% all the time no matter how hard he tried.

Adam started experiencing shortness of breath and angina pain whenever he takes a walk on the street. His blood test showed that his cholesterols (both total cholesterol and LDL cholesterol) were elevated. He was hospitalized for a week and was placed in an intensive care unit. The angiogram test showed the plaque formation in his arteries (what is known as atherosclerosis). His doctor prescribed him a statin drug to lower cholesterols, but that high dosage of statin has been causing him severe muscle pain. When he was in the hospital, some of the nurses recommended him to switch to insulin shots to control his diabetes quickly and effectively. They also recommended him that he could take a diabetes course in his community's diabetes clinic where he lives.

LIFE-CHANGING EVENT TOOK PLACE
When he was 51 years old, Adam attended an insulin-dependant diabetes course in a diabetes clinic, located in his own community. Diabetes clinics are there in every community or hospital to offer hands on training courses on how to inject insulin shots and how to exercise to control diabetes. This diabetes course has changed Adam's life forever. In this diabetes course, an endocrinologist, several nurses and dieticians taught him the following aspects:
- How to inject insulin (both long-acting insulin and rapid-acting insulin) using a syringe and/or a pen,
- How to read labels on any food item to recognize and identify the amount of fat, protein & carbohydrate,
- How to count calories using measuring cups and electronic balance, and by making simple calculations,
- How to determine the amount of carbohydrate present in any meal,
- How to calculate the amount of rapid-acting insulin to be injected for any given meal (1 unit of Humalog insulin is required for 8 grams of carbohydrate),
- How to exercise (either running on a treadmill, biking, or regular walk) in order to lower the after-meal glucose level quickly to normal.

Adam took this course with a great interest, and fully focussed and committed on controlling his type 2 diabetes as quickly as possible. He also read books on diabetes and updated his knowledge in every possible way. He started Method 3 with insulin shots along with exercise, and he successfully controlled his diabetes, and achieved normal hemoglobin A1c level (below 7%) in 6 months.

Believe it or not, it is very easy to control diabetes with insulin shots along with exercise. With Method 3, you can go easy on dietary guidelines and can consume and enjoy high-carbohydrate meals whenever you feel like, and you can still control your diabetes successfully if you can equip your mind with proper knowledge.

The detailed schedule of Adam's diabetes control plan in a typical day, during the past 6 months, is shown below:

7:00 am   Adam wakes up and monitors his fasting blood glucose level early in the morning.
7:05 am   Blood glucose level: 4.8 mmol/L or 86.4 mg/dL.
          He takes coffee with 1% milk, and checks his emails, and listens to music on YouTube video.

7:30 am   He prepares his breakfast, and injects mixed dose of insulin when he is ready to eat.
          (25 units of long-acting insulin Humulin-N, and 8 units of rapid-acting insulin Humalog)

Breakfast (Daily Routine)
7:45 am   BREAKFAST
Adam eats an egg-white omelet (egg-white is one 100% protein) every day in the breakfast. Egg-white omelet is made with veggies (broccoli or cauliflower or spinach, mushrooms, onions, bell peppers with a few drops of extra virgin olive oil), whole wheat bread toasted (no butter added), mustard sauce, a small cup of low-fat yogurt, a small cup of fresh blueberries, and purified water. After the breakfast he goes outside and walks for 10 to 15 minutes and self-monitors his blood glucose level.

8:10 am   Blood glucose level usually at this time of the day : 5.5 mmol/L or 99 mg/dL.

Lunch (Eats Mostly At Home, and Eats Once or Twice a Week in a Restaurant)
11:30 am Adam went to a restaurant to eat lunch today.
Adam eats high-carbohydrate lunch once or twice a week in a restaurant to his fullest satisfaction.

11:45 am Adam injected 20 units of rapid-acting insulin Humalog from his pen,
          and started eating lunch in the restaurant.
LUNCH: Thai cashews chicken cooked with bell peppers, onions, peas & soy sauce, a bowl of white rice, one spring roll, and a glass of wine. After the lunch, he went into a 7-Eleven store, purchased Drumstick ice cream, and ate it.

12:30 pm Adam went to a gym to exercise. He monitored his glucose level again.
          It was 13.8 mmol/L or 248.4 mg/dL.
          Adam ran on a treadmill for 30 minutes, and monitored again.
 1:05 pm Blood glucose level dropped to: 8.5 mmol.L or 153 mg/dL.
 1:10 pm Adam injected 4 more units of rapid-acting insulin Humalog,
          and ran on treadmill for another 30 min, and monitored.
 1:45 pm Blood glucose level further dropped to: 5.2 mmol.L or 93.6 mg/dL. Adam went home.

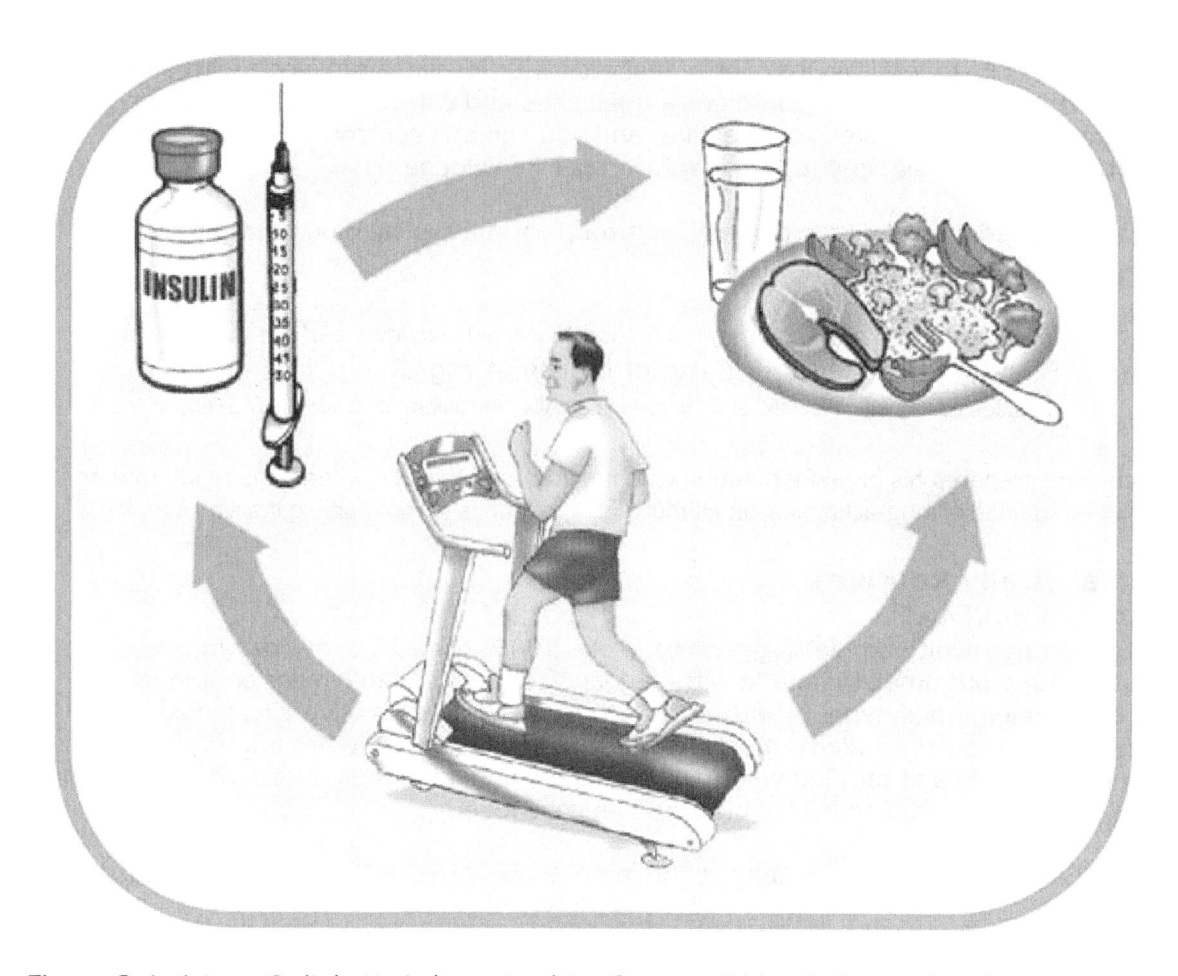

Figure 3.4   A type 2 diabetic is lowering his after-meal blood glucose level
              with the aid of rapid-acting insulin and exercise (Running On a Treadmill).

IMPORTANT POINTS TO REMEMBER
(i) It is important to note here that Adam managed to lower his after-meal spike to perfectly normal within 2 hours after eating a high-carbohydrate meal. Had he not done this, he could have been living with highly elevated blood glucose levels (levels above 20 mmol/L or 360 mg/dL) throughout the afternoon, contributing to elevated average blood glucose level, and in turn elevated hemoglobin A1c. Living like that for months and years could lead to all kinds of long term side effects of chronic and fatal disease called diabetes mellitus.

(ii) Adam injected 20 units of rapid-acting insulin Humalog just before the meal so that his after-meal glucose level would be under 14 mmol/L or 250 mg/dL because he learned that ketones formation occurs if he exercises with blood glucose level over 14 mmol/L or 250 mg/dL. It is important to inject the sufficient amount of rapid-acting insulin Humalog before eating so that your after-meal glucose level would be below 14 mmol/L or 250 mg/dL, and you can exercise without panicking about ketones formation. Ketones formation does not occur to everybody so you should find out if your body is sensitive to Ketones formation and its symptoms. If your body doesn't form ketones, you don't need to worry about this aspect, and can exercise immediately after a major meal consumption even if your after-meal glucose level is more than 14 mmol/L or 250 mg/dL.

2:30 pm   Adam monitored again. Blood glucose level rose to: 9.1 mmol/L or 163.8 mg/dL. Remember! Adam ate white rice in his lunch. White rice digests and raises blood glucose level for a long time.Therefore he injected another 10 units of rapid-acting insulin Humalog again after he came home, and this treatment kept his blood glucose level normal till 6 pm.

Had he eaten brown rice with his lunch, instead of white rice, his diabetes control could have been a lot easier. However, sometimes, you can enjoy white rice if you know how to control your diabetes by injecting more insulin. You can even eat a large bowl of desert as long as you know how to lower your after-meal glucose level to normal.

6:00 pm   Adam monitored just before dinner. Blood glucose level: 6.5 mmol/L or 117 mg/dL.

Dinner (Daily Routine)
6:05 pm   Adam prepares his dinner, and injects mixed dose of insulin when he is ready to eat dinner. He injected 25 units of Humulin-N and 5 units of rapid-acting insulin Humalog.
6:05 pm   Adam eats a low-carbohydrate meal in his dinner that would not raise his blood glucose level too high.
DINNER: Oven-baked fish, steamed vegetables, one slice of bread and one organic apple or organic banana. After eating, he goes out and walks for 10 to 15 minutes to lower his after-meal glucose level.
9:30 pm   Adam monitors just before going to bed.
             Blood glucose level typically: 6.9 mmol.L or 124.2 mg/dL.

In-Between Meal Snacks (Daily Routine)
Adam eats 3 times a day a few items of the following in-between meal snacks:
- Organic green cabbage cooked with onions, carrots, sweet potatoes, yams, fresh garlic & fresh ginger,
- Cottage cheese dry curd (It contains high protein, zero fat, very low carbohydrate, low sodium),
- Low-fat and low-sugar yogurt,
- Boiled chickpeas & boiled kidney beans,
- Kamut Puffs (crunchy and tasty),
- Fruits (organic banana or apple, avocados, pomelo, grape fruit, oranges, grapes, pears, papaya, lemons & limes, etc.),
- Nuts in limited quantities (cashews, blanched almonds, walnuts, peanuts, etc.).

Adam minimizes and consumes only a little sea salt and extra virgin oil in all his meals. Minimization of the salt consumption and oil consumption helps lose weight, and keeps the blood pressure under control.
Whenever he eats a snack, he injects a few units of Humalog insulin so that his blood glucose level remains normal. From his extensive experience on monitoring and controlling, he easily guesses the number of units of Humalog to be injected.

Adam's self-blood glucose monitoring data in a typical day are shown below:
Table 3.10

Time	7:00 AM	8:10 AM	12:30 PM	1:05 PM	1:45 PM	2:30 PM	6:00 PM	9:30 PM	Average	A1c
Glucose (mmol/L)	4.8	5.5	13.8	8.5	5.2	9.1	6.5	6.9	7.5	6.6%
Glucose (mg/dL)	86.4	99	248.4	153	93.6	163.8	117	124.2	135.7	6.6%

Adam calculated his daily average blood glucose level as 7.5 mmol/L or 135.7 mg/dL.
He also determined the hemoglobin A1c (from A1c Chart) as 6.6%.

Adam lost weight by following the dietary guidelines. His arteries are cleared and unclogged.
He doesn't suffer from shortness of breath or angina pain anymore.

He does not need high doses of statin drug anymore so he doesn't suffer from muscle pain.
He takes very low dosage of statin Zocor (5 mg or 10 g), and takes cholesterol-lowering supplement guggul.

His cholesterols are now perfectly normal. Adam is happier than ever.
Adam brought his health back to normal with diligence, knowledge and determination.
Adam has become a self-taught doctor of diabetes control.

EXAMPLE 4: A TYPE 2 DIABETIC HAS BEEN CONTROLLING HIS DIABETES LIKE AN EXPERT

Sam is a 51-year-old Type 2 diabetic. After every major high-carbohydrate meal consumption, his blood glucose level rises above 18 mmol/L o 324 mg/dL. His hemoglobin A1c is over 9.8%. During the past 2 years, he has been experiencing heart disease, angina and kidney disease.
He has been injecting too much insulin (25 units of Humalog) to lower his high blood sugar levels without incorporating exercise along with insulin shots. He has read a lot about diabetes and insulin. He learned that too much insulin stimulates the brain so that a person feels hungry and eats more and also causes the liver to add fat in the belly. He decided to optimize the insulin dose for the evening meal by implementing 1 hour of exercise. His diabetes control strategy is described below with his physical activity in the evening after dinner:

5:30 pm   Prepared a major meal of 900 kilocalories (150 gm of carbohydrate). Skinless chicken cooked with veggies and fat free soy milk, brown rice, sea salt & cayenne pepper.
6:00 pm   Monitored fasting glucose (see table below); consumed major meal.
6:30 pm   Monitored blood glucose level (see table below).
   He learned that he should not exercise if his level is over 13 mmol/L or 234 mg/dL.
   (Ketones formation could occur in the body if he exercises at high glucose levels)
   Injected 6 units of Humalog to bring his level down to 13 mmol/L.
7:00 pm   Blood glucose level dropped to 12.9 mmol/L or 232 mg/dL.
7:00 pm   Injected 4 more units of Humalog, and started walking.
   Walked precisely 7 ½ minutes, carefully looking at his wristwatch.
   Came home by walking another 7 ½ minutes (total 15 minutes).
   Monitored his glucose and spent 5 minutes for record keeping.
   Repeated the same 3 more times to complete 1 hour of exercise.

Table 3.11   ◄--------------- Walked ---------------►

Time	6:00 PM	6:30 PM	7:00 PM	7:15 PM	7:35 PM	7:55 PM	8:15 PM
Glucose (mmol/L)	6	19.4	12.5	8.5	7.6	6.1	4.7
Glucose (mg/dL)	108	349	225	153	136.8	109.8	84.6

For 150 gm of carbohydrate in a meal, it would require 19 units of Humalog (1 unit for every 8 gm). But Ervin lowered his level to normal with 11 units only, cutting Humalog dose by 47%. He has controlled his after-meal glucose levels and minimized his Humalog insulin dose every day diligently for 6 months. His hemoglobin A1c has dropped from 9.8% to 6.7% in 6 months. Sam is now a happy man. He no longer suffers from angina pain from clogged arteries, and his kidney disease disappeared. He now monitors only a few times a day, and still his diabetes is tightly controlled (his hemoglobin A1c level is less than 7%). His own experience on injecting rapid-acting insulin with every meal on a daily basis has helped him master the concept of controlling diabetes. Sam has become a self-taught master of diabetes control.

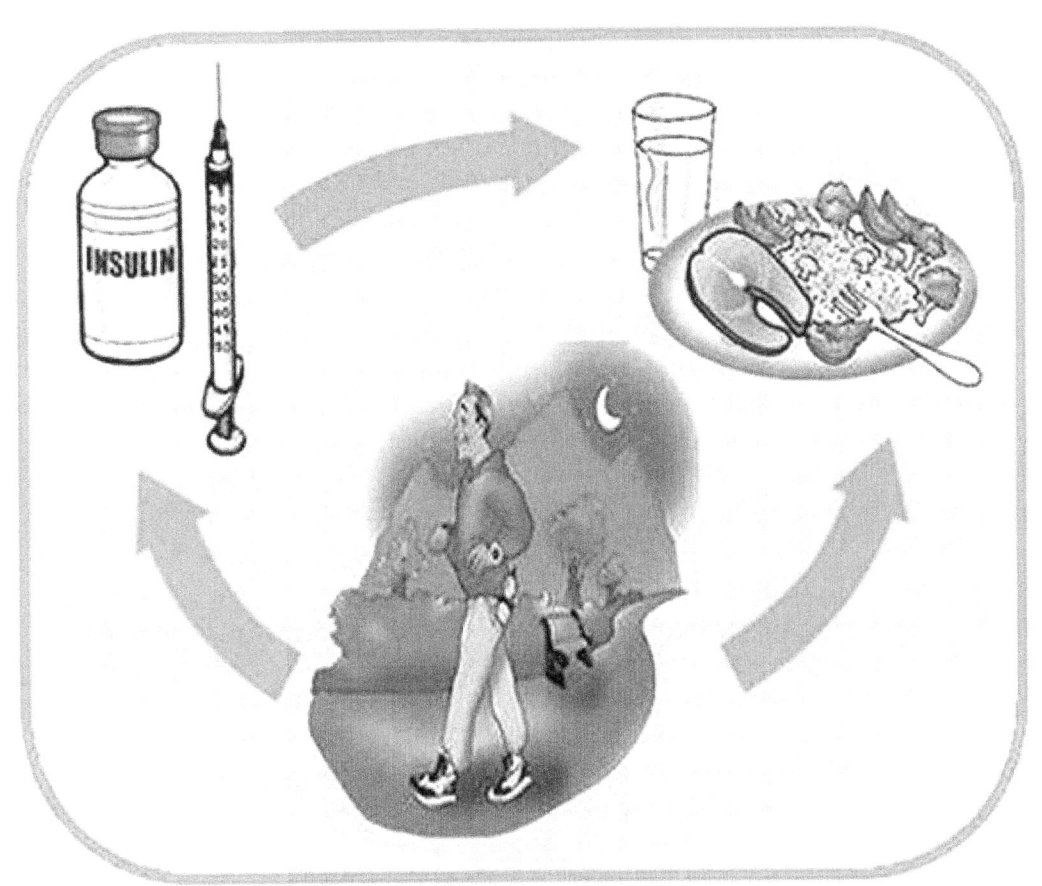

Figure 3.5 A type 2 diabetic is lowering his after-meal blood glucose level with the aid of rapid-acting insulin and exercise (Walking on the Road).

EXAMPLE 5: A TYPE 2 DIABETIC ATHLETE HAS BEEN CONTROLLING HIS DIABETES LIKE AN EXPERT

Ken is a 37-year-old Type 2 diabetic. He is an all-around athlete who exemplifies high achievement in sports, specializing in soccer. He eats in restaurants very often. His blood glucose level reaches over 20 mmol/L or 360 mg/dL after every heavy meal. He does not calculate the insulin dose but guesses how much insulin dose he should inject before and after exercise, with 1 hour of exercise, to keep his glucose level within the normal range. He plays soccer and other games every week¾no problem.

He diligently researched his elevated after-meal blood glucose levels against rapid-acting Humalog doses and exercise through consuming a variety of heavy meals. After a few months, he became a self-taught doctor of diabetes control. Here is a typical example of his one-day activity during his diabetes control plan:

5:15 pm   Went into a restaurant where dinner buffet is served.
          Monitored his fasting blood glucose level (see table below).
          Injected 12 units of insulin with his Humalog pen.
          He has already researched. These 12 units will drop his blood glucose
          level just below 13 mmol/L or 234 mg/dL so that he can exercise.
          Consumed a heavy meal in the restaurant (soup, bread, salad,
          chicken, rice, legumes, baked potato, dessert and beer).
5:50 pm   Went to a gym and monitored his blood glucose (see table below).
6:00 pm   Ran on the treadmill at a speed of 4.0 mph with 1.0 inclination.
          Every 15 minutes, he interrupted treadmill for 5 minutes,
          monitored and recorded his blood glucose (see table below).
          He brought his after-meal glucose level to normal in 1 ½ hours.
7:05 pm   Went into the restroom and took a shower.
7:25 pm   Monitored his glucose level; Increased to 10 mmol/L or 180 mg/dL.
          Injected a second shot, some 5 units of Humalog.
          He knows that this treatment will keep his levels normal till midnight.

Table 3.12

Speed: 4.0 mph; Calories burned: 355 Kcal
◄---------------- Treadmill ------------►

Time	5:15 PM	5:50 PM	6:15 PM	6:25 PM	6:45 PM	7:05 PM
Glucose (mmol/L)	5.3	12.7	10.8	7.5	6.8	5
Glucose (mg/dL)	95.4	228.6	194.4	135	122.4	104.4

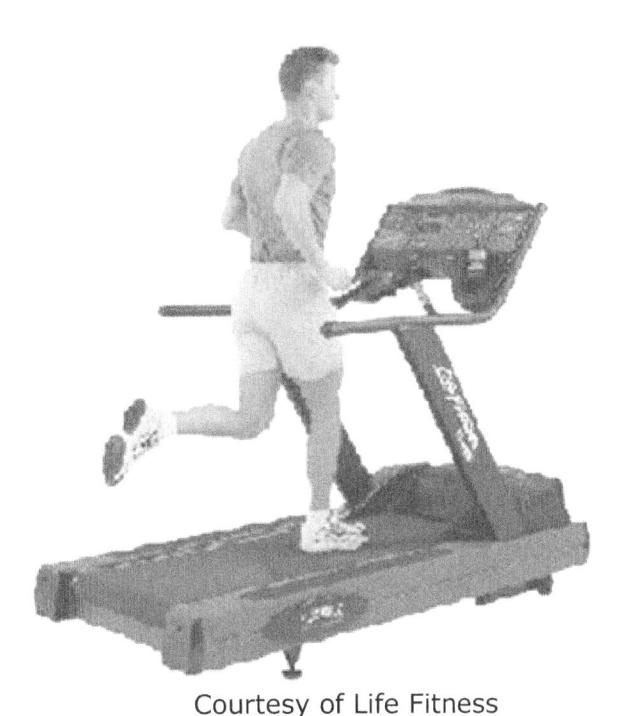

Courtesy of Life Fitness
Figure 3.6 A type 2 diabetic athlete is lowering his after-meal blood glucose level with the aid of rapid-acting insulin and exercise (Running On a Treadmill).

EXAMPLE 6: A TYPE 2 DIABETIC ATHLETE HAS BEEN CONTROLLING HIS DIABETES LIKE AN EXPERT

Anderson, a 52-year-old athletic person, used to be a very active football player and wrestler. Three years ago, he was diagnosed with Type-2 diabetes. Anderson chose to take insulin shots to control his diabetes effectively. Anderson was on his way home driving from Seattle, WA, United States to Vancouver, BC, Canada. It was 5:30 pm. It would take another hour to get home. He was hungry and decided to eat. He drove into a highway restaurant in Bellingham and ate a lot of food from the buffet (salad bar, pasta, chicken, sushi, tempura, fruit salad, dessert and beer). He injected 10 units of Humalog with his insulin pen just before the meal. He finished his meal by 6 pm. He got home at 7 pm, and monitored his blood glucose level. It was very high: 15.5 mmol/L or 279 mg/dL. He wanted to go to the gym and do treadmill. But he had already read the book Permanent Diabetes Control in which he learned that he should not do exercise if his blood glucose level is above 14 mmol/L or 250 mg/dL because ketones would form and accumulate in his body. He therefore injected another shot of Humalog, about 4 units, and drove to the gym in half an hour (7:30 pm), where he monitored his level again as 12.5 mmol/L or 225 mg/dL. He then exercised (ran on treadmill at high speed) for 1 hour, and found his glucose level dropped to 4.9 mmol/L or 88.2 mg/dL by 8:30 pm. He got home by 9 pm and monitored his level again. The level had risen to 8.1 mmol/L or 151.2 mg/dL. He injected another shot, 4 more units of Humalog, and watched TV. By 9:30 am his level had dropped to 5.3 mmol/L or 95 mg/dL and remained normal till 11:45 pm. He then injected 15 units of intermediate-acting insulin Humalog-N, ate fresh carrots and a few dried apricots (bedtime snack), and went to sleep. By 7 am the next morning, his level was 5.5 mmol/L or 98 mg/dL.

Anderson made clear notes on items he consumed in the restaurant and all insulin shots injected so that next time he can consume the same meal and manage his insulin shots comfortably. He eats in the restaurant to his fullest satisfaction twice a week, and his diabetes is still tightly controlled.

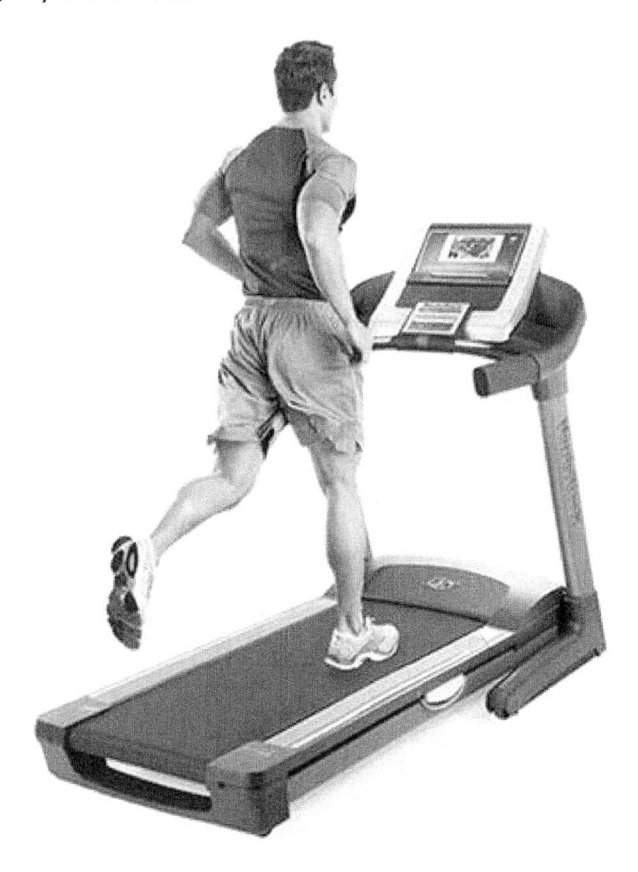

Courtesy of Life Fitness
Figure 3.7 A type 2 diabetic athlete is lowering his after-meal blood glucose level with the aid of rapid-acting insulin and exercise (Running On a Treadmill).

Example 7: A LADY WITH TYPE 2 DIABETES HAS BEEN CONTROLLING HER DIABETES LIKE AN EXPERT

Elza is a 64-year-old female. She has been Type 2 diabetic for 15 years and switched to insulin shots 2 to 3 years ago. She lives in New Westminster, BC, Canada, where she knew a restaurant called "Old Spaghetti Factory." She is cautious with her health and has been practicing diabetes control for the past 2 to 3 years. She ordered a Spaghetti meal in the restaurant brought it home at 5:15 pm. She separated all the meal items: baked chicken, spaghetti, soup, garlic bread, lettuce, tomatoes, and measured the weight of each item. From the calorie-counter tables, she noted the breakdown of fat, protein and carbohydrate for spaghetti, soup, garlic bread, lettuce and tomatoes (chicken has no carbohydrate). From the weight of each item, she calculated the carbohydrate content of each item, and added them up to obtain total carbohydrate content of her meal as approximately 150 g. She knew that 1 unit of Humalog is needed for 8 g of carbohydrate. So for 150 g of carbohydrate, she needed 19 units of Humalog. Because she planned to exercise, her insulin dose required was 9.5 units (half of 19 units). She injected 10 units of Humalog just before she ate at 5:30 pm. Her level rose to 12.6 mmol/L or 226.8 mg/dL 30 minutes after the meal. She walked for 1 hour in her neighborhood. She monitored her levels every half an hour. After 1 hour of walking, her blood glucose level dropped to 5.5 mmol/L or 102.6 mg/dL. She then injected a second shot, about 5.8 units of Humalog. Her levels remained normal until midnight. She then took 15 units of Humulin-N, ate one Savory Garlic Matzo (fat free and cholesterol free) and baby carrots as her bedtime snack, and went to sleep. By next morning, her level was 4.6 mmol/L or 82.8 mg/dL (perfectly normal).

Next time when she goes to the same restaurant (Old Spaghetti Factory), she can sit and eat in the restaurant without panicking, inject 19 units of Humalog, and eat the Spaghetti meal and still keep her after-meal blood glucose level normal . Or if she is planning to walk after the meal, she could cut the Humalog dose in half, inject it and eat the meal, and walk afterwards. She can order the same meal and inject 5.8 units of Humalog twice (before meal and after exercise). Elza mastered the concept of diabetes control with insulin and exercise. Her hemoglobin A1c has been normal (under 7%) for the past 2 to 3 years. Her diabetes has been permanently controlled, as she mastered the topic. She doesn't need any doctors to take care of her health, except for blood test requisitions and prescriptions. Elza has become an expert of diabetes control.

HOW TO CONTROL TYPE 1 DIABETES WITH INSULIN SHOTS & EXERCISE

The diabetes control for type 1 diabetes or type 2 diabetes remains exactly the same.
A type 1 diabetic person needs more insulin dosages than a type 2 diabetic person. For type 2 diabetic or type 1 diabetic, insulin dosages vary from person to person and from meal to meal. Each person is different. Each person (either type 1 or type 2 diabetic) should use his/her own insulin dosages. But in terms of controlling diabetes, the method remains the same.

Refer to preceding examples. And suppose that the person in those examples is type 1 diabetic, and controlling his/her type 1 diabetes. Lifestyle changes (dietary guidelines), insulin shots, exercise program, and managing type 1 diabetes remain the same.

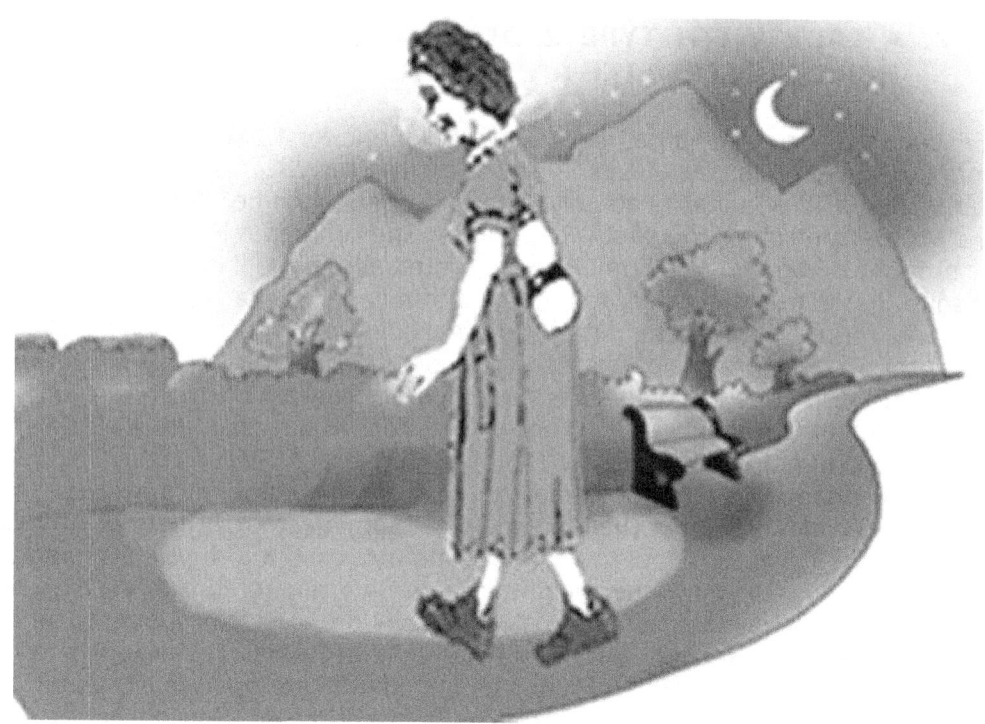

Figure 3.8 A type 2 diabetic is lowering her after-meal blood glucose level with the aid of rapid-acting insulin and exercise (Walking on the Road).

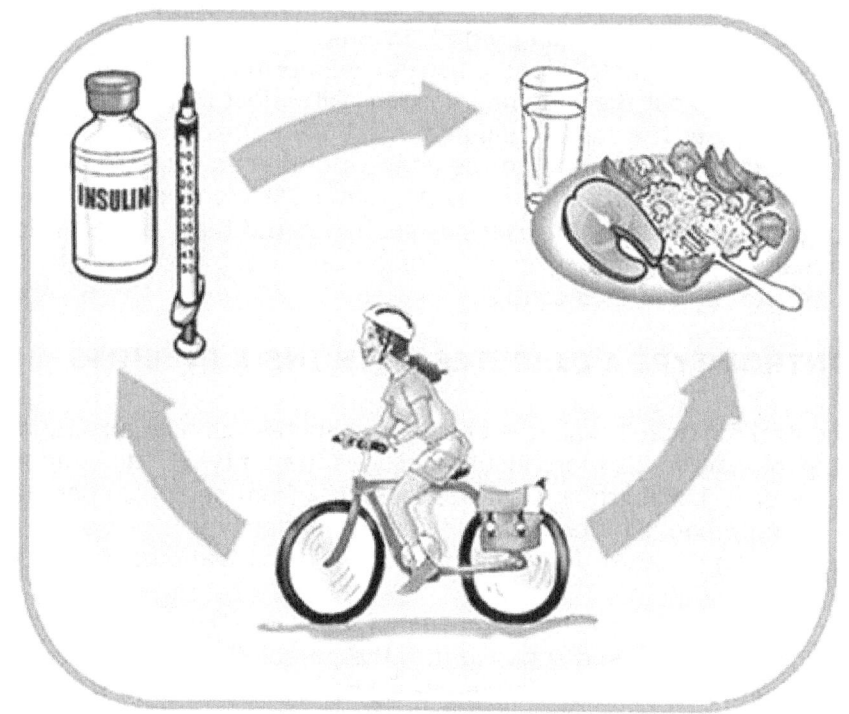

Figure 3.9 A type 1 diabetic is lowering her after-meal blood glucose level with the aid of rapid-acting insulin and exercise (Cycling on the Road).

ADVANTAGES OF METHOD 3 (WITH INSULIN SHOTS)
There is no such disadvantage in terms of controlling diabetes using Method 3.

- You don't really need to worry about high self-discipline and high willpower. You can go easy on dietary changes as long as you know how to take insulin shots before or after every meal consumption (breakfast, lunch, dinner and all snacks). However, a healthy lifestyle is extremely important for a diabetic person. Eating out a high-carbohydrate meal in a restaurant once or twice a week is okay as long you master the concept of controlling the after-meal spike immediately after the consumption.
- You can enjoy a large high-carbohydrate meal by eating in a buffet-serving restaurant, including a large bowl of desert, and can lower your after-meal glucose spike to normal, within 1 or 2 hours, if you know how to do it correctly by injecting the right amount of insulin, accompanied by an after-meal exercise.
- A highly knowledgeable diabetic person can very easily lower his/her steep blood glucose spike to perfectly normal in 30 to 60 minutes by injecting the right amount of insulin and by running on a treadmill. Even a simple walking exercise on the road with insulin injected would lower the steep glucose spike.
- It is the best method to achieve perfect diabetes control when your body produces a little or no insulin.
- You can see immediate results, and achieve perfect control for the rest of your life if you master the subject matter.
- Perfect diabetes control is not possible with pills (oral medications). When you are on pills and consume a large amount of high-carbohydrate meal and are faced by a steep glucose spike, there is nothing you can do about it, but wait until the next morning to see normal fasting glucose level. Whereas with rapid-acting insulin & exercise, you can immediately lower your after-meal blood glucose spike, and can keep your A1c level normal.

DISADVANTAGES OF METHOD 3 (WITH INSULIN SHOTS)

- Some people are scared and don't feel comfortable to deal with needles every day because they are not accustomed to needles. They don't realize the fact that they can very easily learn how to inject insulin shots in order to lower the after-meal spike by taking a hands on course in any diabetic clinic in their community.

- Other than that, rapid-acting insulin (such as Humalog) along with exercise is the best treatment to control diabetes, it doesn't matter whether you are either type 2 diabetic or types 1 diabetic. Try it out!

WHY SHOULD THE INSULIN DOSE BE OPTIMIZED?

Evening meal or any major meal causes the highest blood glucose levels in people with diabetes. Elevated blood glucose levels are accumulated in the bloodstream soon after the major meal consumption, dominate in and largely contribute to establishing the average blood glucose level in 90 days.

Hemoglobin A1c is a parameter that directly reveals the degree of "diabetes control" during the preceding 90 days. Red blood cells live in the bloodstream 60 to 90 days. Every 90 days, new red blood cells are born. Hemoglobin is a protein molecule that carries and supplies oxygen from the lungs to the trillions of body's cells wherever it is needed. While the blood circulates, depending on how high or how low the blood glucose level is, a certain amount of glucose is attached to the hemoglobin molecules to form glycated hemoglobin. Different people call it with different names: glycated A1c, hemoglobin A1c (HbA1c), or simply A1c. Therefore, by measuring the hemoglobin A1c level in a laboratory from the patient's blood sample, it is possible to know the average blood glucose level and the degree to which it has been controlled over the preceding 90 days. The hemoglobin A1c chart was developed to show the influence of average blood glucose level in 90 days versus hemoglobin A1c.

From this A1c chart, one can firmly confirm that elevated average blood glucose level indicates the elevated hemoglobin A1c. Elevated hemoglobin A1c means the diabetes has been poorly controlled. Therefore elevated after-meal glucose levels must be slashed as quickly as possible and brought to normal within 1 or 2 hour of the major meal consumption in order to bring hemoglobin A1c close to its normal value. Normal hemoglobin A1c means the diabetes has been tightly controlled.

WHY SHOULD THE INSULIN DOSE BE OPTIMIZED?

The artificial insulin dose must be optimized (and minimized), because too much insulin causes hypoglycemia and constricts arteries leading to heart attack and coronary heart disease. Too much insulin also stimulates the brain so that a person feels hungry and eats more and causes the liver to manufacture fat in the belly. Too little insulin on the other hand is not enough to cover the entire meal and to maintain normal glucose levels. An optimum insulin dose is therefore crucial. Insulin is synthesized in such a way that it starts flowing and working a lot more quickly and much more effectively with exercise.
A continuous exercise (30 to 60 minutes), either treadmill, biking or regular walk, should be introduced into the diabetes control plan in order to lower after-meal glucose level, burn fat, lose calories, and optimize both insulin dose and insulin action. If the exercise is introduced immediately after every heavy meal, it not only minimizes the insulin dose but in addition maximizes insulin action and prevents after-meal glucose levels from rising too high, thereby keeping the diabetes under tight control. The following procedures are being recommended by Dr. RK to optimize the insulin dose.

HOW TO OPTIMIZE THE INSULIN DOSE BY TRIAL AND ERROR PROCEDURE?

A diabetic person, before using the method described here, should have undergone an insulin-dependant diabetes course in a local diabetes clinic in his/her area. In this hands on course, they teach the following aspects:

- How to inject insulin (both long-acting insulin and rapid-acting insulin) using a syringe and/or a pen,
- How to read labels on any food item to recognize and identify the amount of fat, protein & carbohydrate,

- How to count calories using measuring cups and electronic balance, and by making simple calculations,
- How to determine the amount of carbohydrate present in any meal,
- How to calculate the amount of rapid-acting insulin to be injected for any given meal (1 unit of Humalog insulin is required for 8 grams of carbohydrate),
- How to exercise (either running on a treadmill, biking, or regular walk) in order to lower the after-meal glucose level quickly to normal.

A diabetic person should have a clear knowledge on the amount of carbohydrate content of a food item and/or a meal being consumed, and should be able to guess the insulin dose. With experience, over time, this guessing of insulin dose becomes an easy and enjoyable task.

TRIAL AND ERROR PROCEDURE: SIMPLIFIED APPROACH DIABETES COBTROL

a. Small Meal

Example: It could be a brown toast with 2 hash brown patties and a small cup of apple juice, and a coffee with 1% milk.

- Inject 5 units of rapid-acting insulin Humalog just before eating.
- Consume the meal, and start exercising (Just go out and walk) for 15 to 20 minutes. Or, if you have a bike at home, ride the bike.
- Monitor blood glucose level. It should be close to normal.
   Normal: 5 mmol/L or 90 mg/dL
- If the glucose level reached normal, you have done your job.
- If the glucose level did not reach normal, then inject a few more units of rapid-acting insulin Humalog so that the level would reach normal.
- Your goal is to lower your after-meal glucose level to normal as quickly as possible within 30 minutes, by guessing the insulin dose by trial and error.
- This experience will help you inject insulin more precisely from next day.

b. Mid-Sized Meal

Example: It could be a whole wheat bagel served with cream cheese, a soup and baked potatoes, and a herbal tea.
- Inject 10 units of rapid-acting insulin Humalog just before eating.
- Consume the meal, and start exercising (Just go out and walk) for 30 minutes. Or, if you have a bike at home, ride the bike.
- Monitor blood glucose level. It should be close to normal.
   Normal: 5 mmol/L or 90 mg/dL
- If the glucose level reached normal, you have done your job.
- If the glucose level did not reach normal, then inject 5 more units of rapid-acting insulin Humalog so that the level would reach normal.
- Monitor after 30 minutes. If the glucose level did not reach normal, then inject a few more units of rapid-acting insulin Humalog so that the level would reach normal.
- Your goal is to lower your after-meal glucose level to normal as quickly as possible within an hour, by guessing the insulin dose by trial and error.
- This experience will help you inject insulin more precisely from next day.

c. Large Meal (Low Carbohydrate)

It could be a large, carefully prepared low-carbohydrate meal consumed at home by following dietary guidelines.

Example: Baked skinless chicken, brown rice, steamed legumes and veggies, and a fruit.

LOW INSULIN DOSE & EXERCISE REQUIRED
- Guess insulin dose, inject first shot, eat, exercise 60 min & monitor.
- Your blood glucose level should have been dropped to normal by now!
- Inject second shot to prevent it from rising
  (some people don't need second shot).
- The amount of insulin varies from person to person & from meal to meal.
- Each person needs to determine his/her own insulin dose for a meal.

- Inject 10 units of rapid-acting insulin Humalog just before eating.
- Consume the meal, and start exercising (Treadmill, Biking or Walking)
  for 60 minutes. Or, if you have a bike at home, ride the bike for 60 minutes.
- Monitor blood glucose level, and check if it reached normal.
- If the blood glucose level is not normal, inject more insulin & monitor.
- This approach would keep your glucose level normal up to 6 hours.
- This experience will help you inject insulin more precisely from next day.

d. Large Meal (High Carbohydrate)

Example: It could be a large high-carbohydrate meal consumed in a restaurant to the fullest satisfaction. Or it could be a large unlimited meal consumed in a buffet-serving restaurant. Refer to Example 2 in which Adam ate lunch (a large meal) in a Thai restaurant, and exercised to lower his after-meal glucose level to normal.

HIGH INSULIN DOSE & EXERCISE REQUIRED
- Guess insulin dose, inject first shot, eat, exercise 30 min & monitor.
- Guess insulin dose, inject second shot, exercise 30 min & monitor.
- Guess insulin dose, inject third shot, no exercise & monitor.
- Your blood glucose level should have been dropped to normal by now!
- This procedure varies from person to person & from meal to meal.
- Each person needs to determine his/her own insulin dose for a meal.

- Inject 10 units of rapid-acting insulin Humalog just before eating.
- Consume the meal, and start exercising (Treadmill, Biking or Walking)
  for 30 minutes. Or, if you have a bike at home, ride the bike for 30 minutes.
- Monitor blood glucose level, and check if it reached normal.
            Normal: 5 mmol/L or 90 mg/dL
- If the glucose level did not reach normal, then inject 5 more units of
  Humalog, and continue exercise for another 30 minutes.
- Monitor blood glucose level. It should be close to normal.
- After 30 minutes, monitor again. You will find the glucose level risen.
- Then inject more insulin (5 to 10 units depending on the glucose level).
- After 30 minutes, monitor again. You will find the glucose level normal.
- This approach would keep your glucose level normal up to 6 hours.
- This experience will help you inject insulin more precisely from next day.

Refer to Example 3 in which Adam consumed a large high-carbohydrate lunch in a restaurant including a cup of white rice and ice cream to his fullest satisfaction, and injected rapid-acting insulin Humalog 2 to 3 times, and brought his after-meal glucose level to normal in 2 hours, just by guessing the insulin dose by trial and error.

   Adam injected Humalog 3 times for the large meal he consumed:
   20 units + 4 unit + 10 units = 34 units

If Adam did not exercise, he could have needed to inject more than twice that amount (more than 68 units) of rapid-acting insulin to lower his after-meal glucose level to normal. And that excess amount of insulin could have stimulated the Adam's brain to feel hungry, eat more, and could have caused his liver to manufacture fat in the belly, leading to a disastrous performance. Therefore it is obvious that the rapid-acting insulin dose must be optimized by introducing exercise into the diabetes control plan.

TRIAL AND ERROR PROCEDURE: DIABETES CONTROL SOPHISTICATED APPROACH

Please see next page for the flow sheet of trial and error procedure.

Rapid-acting insulin dose for any given meal can be precisely determined by following the trial and error procedure steps described in the following flow sheet. The amount of insulin determined through this trial and error procedure varies from person to person & from meal to meal. Every diabetic person needs to determine his/her own optimal insulin dose for a given meal.

WHY ARE AFTER-MEAL BLOOD GLUCOSE LEVELS NOT TOO HIGH? AN IMPORTANT CLARIFICATION

By examining the self-blood glucose monitoring results in Method 1, Method 2, Method 3, a reader might wonder and raise a question such as "why are the after-meal blood glucose levels not significantly high enough?". Most of the data showed in these examples have after meal-glucose levels under 13 mmol/L or 234 mg/dL. To understand this, please refer to Method 3 where "Ketones Formation" and "Ketoacidosis" are explained. A diabetic person should be cautious beforehand and should not exercise when the after-meal glucose levels are higher than 13 mmol/L or 234 mg/dL, unless the exercise suits his/her body without forming ketones. A diabetic person should inject the correct amount of insulin just before consuming a major meal to lower his/her blood glucose level close to 13 mmol/L or 234 mg/dL, and then exercise in order to lower his/her after-meal blood glucose level to perfectly normal (5 mmol/L or 90 md/dL). That is why in all the self-blood glucose monitoring data, you will find the after-meal blood glucose levels below 13 mmol/L or 234 mg/dL.

TRIAL AND ERROR PROCEDURE: DIABETES CONTROL
HOW TO DETERMINE THE INSULIN DOSE TO LOWER AFTER-MEAL GLUCOE LEVEL TO NORMAL
Developed by Rao Konduru, PhD

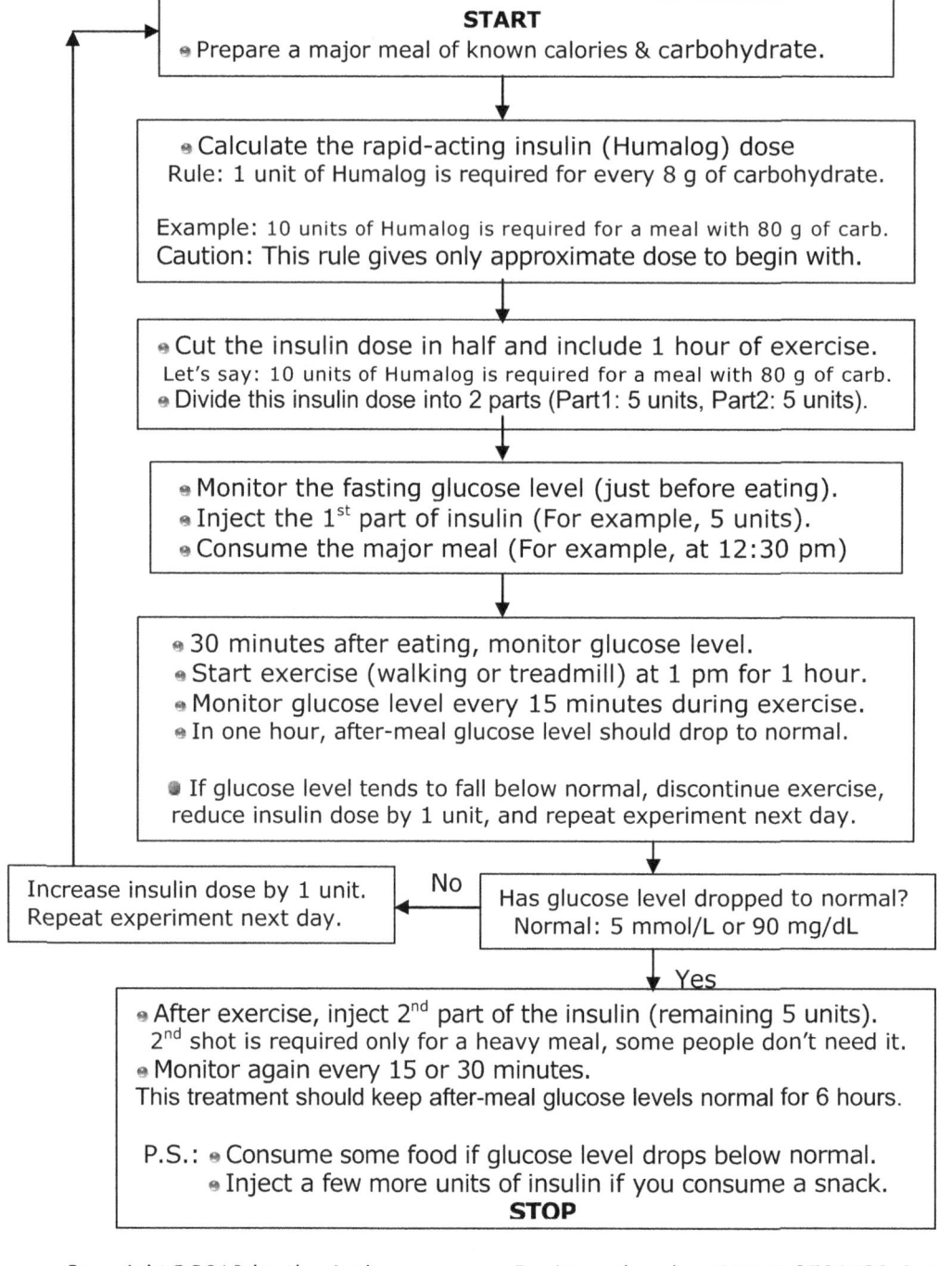

START
- Prepare a major meal of known calories & carbohydrate.

- Calculate the rapid-acting insulin (Humalog) dose
Rule: 1 unit of Humalog is required for every 8 g of carbohydrate.

Example: 10 units of Humalog is required for a meal with 80 g of carb.
Caution: This rule gives only approximate dose to begin with.

- Cut the insulin dose in half and include 1 hour of exercise.
Let's say: 10 units of Humalog is required for a meal with 80 g of carb.
- Divide this insulin dose into 2 parts (Part1: 5 units, Part2: 5 units).

- Monitor the fasting glucose level (just before eating).
- Inject the 1st part of insulin (For example, 5 units).
- Consume the major meal (For example, at 12:30 pm)

- 30 minutes after eating, monitor glucose level.
- Start exercise (walking or treadmill) at 1 pm for 1 hour.
- Monitor glucose level every 15 minutes during exercise.
- In one hour, after-meal glucose level should drop to normal.

- If glucose level tends to fall below normal, discontinue exercise, reduce insulin dose by 1 unit, and repeat experiment next day.

Has glucose level dropped to normal?
Normal: 5 mmol/L or 90 mg/dL

No → Increase insulin dose by 1 unit. Repeat experiment next day.

Yes ↓

- After exercise, inject 2nd part of the insulin (remaining 5 units).
  2nd shot is required only for a heavy meal, some people don't need it.
- Monitor again every 15 or 30 minutes.
This treatment should keep after-meal glucose levels normal for 6 hours.

P.S.: - Consume some food if glucose level drops below normal.
      - Inject a few more units of insulin if you consume a snack.

STOP

Copyright©2019 by the Author   Registered under ISBN 0-9731120-0-X

Dr. RK'S DIABETES HAS BEEN PERMANENTLY CONTROLLED

After suffering from a sudden heart attack in 1998, even though his left artery was 75% clogged and he could not walk a block due to severe angina pain, Dr. RK said "NO" to bypass surgery. He did what none of us would even think of doing. He simply relied on his natural self-prevention diet and exercise, and with it "reversed his critical diabetic heart disease in a matter of months", and developed a method to accomplish Permanent Diabetes Control. He proved to the medical community that a bypass surgery is unnecessary in most cases. He also came up with a trial and error procedure to determine the optimal insulin dose that would tightly control diabetes in 90 days, and would allow a diabetic person to live like a normal person for the rest of his/her life.

Please see his official blood test results below, and notice that his hemoglobin A1c level dropped from a high-risk 12% to a stunning 6.2%, 5.5%, 5.2%, 5.0%, and has been under 6% consistently for many years. His personal best hemoglobin A1c level of 5% is an extraordinary result any diabetic person would hope to accomplish in a lifetime. In spite of being seriously diabetic person and highly insulin-dependent, Dr. RK accomplished Permanent Diabetes Control with his own diligence and expert knowledge on diabetes. Perhaps he is the only diabetic person living in this world with Permanent Diabetes Control!

Official Blood Text Results of Controlled Diabetes

Listed below are the official blood test results of Dr. RK, performed with a physician's requisition, by BC Biomedical Laboratories (Currently Life Labs), Vancouver, British Columbia, Canada.

Table 3.13

Date	Fasting Glucose	Fasting Glucose	Hemoglobin A1c
Units	mmol/L	mg/dL	g/g Hgb (%)
Normal	(3.6 - 6.1)	(65 – 110)	4.5% - 6.2%
11-Jun-1997			**12.0%**
18-Mar-1998	Suffered Heart Attack (not controlled until 1998)!		
21-Apr-1998	9.2	165.6	9.6%
26-Oct-1998	5.7	102.6	8.0%
22-Jan-1999	6.0	108.0	8.4%
05-May-1999	5.1	91.8	8.1%
07-Jan-2000	7.0	126.0	10.2%
07-Jun-2000	Started controlling diabetes seriously!		
01-Aug-2000	6.0	108.0	8.2%
19-Sep-2000	5.6	100.8	7.4%
19-Jan-2001	4.9	88.2	6.6%
29-Non-2001	5.2	93.6	6.5%
05-Mar-2002	5.2	93.6	6.6%
06-May-2002	4.9	88.2	6.5%
26-Jun-2002	4.4	79.2	6.6%
02-Oct-2002	4.0	72.0	6.3%
30-Jan-2003	5.1	91.8	6.2%
08-Apr-2003	4.7	84.6	6.2%

Date	Fasting Glucose	Fasting Glucose	Hemoglobin A1c
Units	mmol/L	mg/dL	g/g Hgb (%)
Normal	(3.6 - 6.1)	(65 – 110)	4.5% - 6.2%
03-Aug-2011	4.9	88.2	6.0%
01-Nov-2011	3.9	70.2	5.8%
01-Feb-2012	3.9	70.2	5.5%
01-May-2012	4.4	79.2	5.5%
01-Aug-2012	3.7	66.7	5.5%
23-Oct-2012	4.1	73.8	5.5%
17-Jan-2013	4.3	77.4	5.3%
01-May-2013	2.9	52.2	5.6%
21-Aug-2013	5.1	91.8	5.5%
02-Jan-2014	4.2	75.8	5.8%
01-Apr-2014	4.0	72.0	5.9%
02-Jul-2014	4.7	84.8	5.7%
01-Oct-2014	3.6	64.8	5.5%
02-Jan-2015	4.9	88.2	5.4%
01-Apr-2015	4.7	84.8	5.4%
03-Jul-2015	5.3	84.8	5.6%
01-Oct-2015	4.1	73.8	5.8%
02-Jan-2016	5.7	102.6	5.8%
01-Apr-2016	4.4	79.2	5.6%
02-Jul-2016	5.5	99.0	5.9%
01-Oct-2016	5.3	95.4	5.0%
			Personal Best
05-Jan-2017	5.1	91.8	5.6%
02-Apr-2017	5.5	99.0	5.4%
02-Jul-2017	4.5	81.0	5.6%
02-Jan-2018	4.2	75.6	5.7%
03-Apr-2018	4.8	86.4	5.9%
02-Jul-2018	4.6	82.8	5.7%
01-Oct-2018	3.4	61.2	5.7%
02-Jan-2019	4.7	84.8	5.5%
01-Apr-2019	3.9	70.2	5.6%
30-Jun-2019	4.2	85.6	5.5%
01-Oct-2019	4.8	86.4	5.6%

CLOSING REMARKS

If you master the concept of injecting rapid-acting insulin along with exercise, you can go easy on the dietary guidelines, and enjoy a high-carbohydrate meal (your favorite meal in a restaurant) once or twice a week. Some diabetic people with expert knowledge go easy on the dietary guidelines and still manage to control diabetes with insulin shots, keep their A1c perfectly normal, and live like a normal person (these people with expert knowledge know how to inject the right amount of rapid-acting insulin, by trial and error and exercise, and lower after-meal blood glucose spike quickly to normal, and know how to achieve normal A1c).

With experience, over time, it becomes very easy to control diabetes with insulin! You cannot do that with oral medications. If you are type 2 diabetic, and currently on pills, and living with uncontrolled diabetes, you need to evaluate your situation. It is strongly recommended to switch to insulin shots. An insulin-dependent type 2 diabetic can control his/her diabetes easily and achieve a perfect normal A1c level in a short period of time, and keep it controlled forever!

What is "Permanent Diabetes Control"?

When a highly knowledgeable diabetic person is living with tightly controlled diabetes for an extended period of time, and is determined to control diabetes forever, his/her diabetes is said to be permanently controlled.

The author of this book (Dr. RK) accomplished "Permanent Diabetes Control" after conducting very many diligent experiments related to diabetic research. He has researched on his own body with chronic diabetes, and studied extensively the combined influence of healthy diet, rapid-acting insulin (Humalog) and after-meal exercise on after-meal blood glucose levels. All that diabetic research information of "Real-Life Case Study" is explained in the next chapter titled "Permanent Diabetes Control".

REFERENCES

1. Permanent Diabetes Control (Book), Subtitle: The Complete Guide to Living Like A Normal Person Forever, Authored by Rao Konduru, MS, PhD, Reviewed and Endorsed by Dr. Marshal Dahl, MD, PhD., Endocrinologist, Faculty of Medicine, University of British Columbia, Vancouver, British Columbia, Canada, First Published in 2003. www.mydiabetescontrol.com

2. The Secret to Controlling Type 2 Diabetes, Subtitle: Addendum to Permanent Diabetes Control, Authored by Rao Konduru, Published in 2019, ISBN # 9780973112054, Available on Amazon.com, www.mydiabetescontrol.com

3. Krall, L.P, MD, and Beaser, R.S, MD, Joslin Diabetes Manual, Philadelphia, Lea and Febiger, Pages 3-6, 135, 138, 1989.

4. Glucose Ranges in People Without Diabetes, Lifescan's One Touch Profile Blood Glucose Monitoring Manual, Table on Page 51, Lifescan, Printed in USA, 1996.

5. Do I Need a Longer Insulin Needle? This question was answered by Christy L. Parkin, MSN, RN, CDE, Diabetes Forecast, The Healthy Living Magazine, 2019. http://www.diabetesforecast.org/2013/dec/do-i-need-a-longer-insulin.html

If you want to read all 12 Chapters, please purchase
PERMANENT DIABETES CONTROL
TABLE OF CONTENTS
Please visit www.mydiabetescontrol.com, and click on "Table of Contents".

	Page
▸ Testimonials	i
▸ Foreword	1
▸ Copyright Page	2
▸ Table of Contents	3

	Page
CHAPTER 1: DIABETES FACTS & STATISTICS	9
▸ Around the World	11
▸ In the USA	12
▸ In Canada	13
▸ Diabetes Statistics Resulted from Heart Disease	14
▸ Good News	14
○ REFERENCES	15

	Page
CHAPTER 2: OVERVIEW OF DIABETES	17
▸ How Glucose Builds Up In the Bloodstream?	19
▸ Diabetes and Pancreas	20
▸ Exocrine Function & Endocrine Function of Pancreas	21
▸ YouTube Videos About Pancreas	23
▸ The Production of Insulin in the Human Body	23
▸ Causes of Diabetes	23
▸ Symptoms of Diabetes	24
▸ Hyperglycemia Versus Hypoglycemia	24
▸ Reasons Why You Have Uncontrolled Diabetes	25
▸ Long Term Complications (Side Effects) of Diabetes	26
▸ Types of Diabetes	26
▸ Medical Check-Up and Diagnosis	28
▸ Self-Blood Glucose Monitoring Devices	29
▸ Continuous Glucose Monitoring Devices (Dexcom & FreeStyle)	30
▸ Routine Tests for Diabetics	31
▸ How Is Blood Glucose Level Expressed for Diabetes?	32
▸ Why Is the Glucose Conversion Factor 18?	32
▸ Normal Blood Glucose Levels and Normal & A1c Level	33
▸ An Example of Diabetes Control	33
○ REFERENCES	34

	Page
● CHAPTER 3: DIABETES CONTROL [A Very Important Chapter if You Are Diabetic]	35
● DIABETES CONTROL BASICS	37
▶ Introduction to Diabetes Control	37
▶ Control Your Diabetes in 90 Days: Why 90 Days?	38
▶ Hemoglobin A1c & Hemoglobin A1c Chart Explained	38
▶ Normal Blood Glucose Levels & Normal Hemoglobin A1c Levels	40
▶ The Secret to Controlling Diabetes Successfully	40
▶ Example 1 & Example 2 to Understand the Secret	41
▶ Can the Hemoglobin A1c Be Determined At Home?	41
▶ How to Calculate Daily Average Blood Glucose Level?	43
▶ WHO CAN USE ORAL MEDICATIONS & WHO CAN USE INSULIN SHOTS?	45
● HOW TO CONTROL DIABETES	46
● METHOD 1: Type 2 Diabetes Control With **Healthy Diet & Exercise (No Medication)**	47
▶ Dietary Guidelines	47
▶ Physical Activity Stimulates the Insulin Production from Pancreas	48
▶ EXAMPLE 1: How to Control Type 2 Diabetes With Healthy Diet, Daily Exercise & Self-Discipline!	48
▶ Disadvantages of Method 1	50
● METHOD 2: Type 2 Diabetes Control With **Healthy Diet, Oral Medication & Exercise**	51
▶ Dietary Guidelines & Oral Medication	51
▶ Physical Activity Stimulates the Insulin Production from Pancreas	52
▶ EXAMPLE 2: How to Control Type 2 Diabetes With Healthy Diet, Oral Medication, Daily Exercise & Self-Discipline!	52
▶ Disadvantages of Method 2	54
● METHOD 3: Type 2 Or Type 1 Diabetes Control With **Healthy Diet, Insulin Shots & Exercise**	57
▶ Introduction	57
▶ Uncontrolled Diabetes Is Dangerous	57
▶ Insulin Is The Best Medication For Diabetes	57
▶ Important Note On Insulin	58
▶ Dietary Guidelines & Rapid-Acting Insulin	58
▶ Physical Activity Stimulates the Insulin Production from Pancreas	59
▶ Physical Activity Also Stimulates the Artificial Insulin Injected	60
▶ How Much Artificial Insulin Is to be Injected?	60
▶ Physical Activity Cuts Insulin Dose In Half	60
▶ Hands On Training Course In A Diabetes Clinic	61
▶ FIVE IMPORTANT PRECAUTIONS	61

		Page
▸ How to Achieve Normal A1c With Insulin Shots & Exercise?		64
• How to Enjoy High Carbohydrate Meals & Slash After-Meal Glucose Spikes?		64
• FIVE EXAMPLES DISCUSSED WITH DAILY DIABETES CONTROL ROUTINE		64
• Example 3, Example 4, Example 5, Example 6, Example 7		64
▸ Advantages of Method 3		75
▸ Disadvantages of Method 3		75
▸ Why Should the Insulin Dose Be Optimized?		76
▸ How to Optimize Insulin Dose by Trial & Error?		76
▸ Trial & Error Procedure: Simplified Approach		77
• For A Small Meal, Mid-Sized Meal & Large Meal		
▸ Trial & Error Procedure: Sophisticated Approach		79
▸ Trial & Error Procedure: Diabetes Control (Flow Sheet)		80
▸ Dr. RK's Diabetes Has Been Controlled Permanently		81
▸ Official Blood Test Results of the Controlled Diabetes		81
▸ CLOSING REMARKS		83
▸ WHAT IS PERMANENT DIABETES CONTROL?		83
○ REFERENCES		83

		Page
• **CHAPTER 4: PERMANENT DIABETES CONTROL**		85
▸ Introduction to REAL-LIFE CASE STUDY		87
▸ Rotation of Injection Sites & Finger Poking Strategy		88
▸ Data Collection and Research (Insulin, Food & Exercise)		90
▸ Influence of Insulin & Exercise On After-Meal Glucose Levels		90
▸ Interpretation of Diabetic Research Results		91
▸ Trial and Error Procedure: Diabetes Control		93
▸ Diabetes Treatment Plan Summarized		94
▸ Humalog Versus Humulin-R		95
▸ Conclusions and Observations		95
▸ Recommendations and Further Study		97
▸ Why do We Have to Do This Way?		97
• **Real-Life Case Study of the Participant (Summary)**		98
• Brief History of the Diabetic Person		98
• Official Blood Test Results: Fasting Glucose & Hemoglobin A1c		99
• Official Blood Test Results of Cholesterols		100
• Up-to-Date Official Blood Test Results of the Participant		102
▸ FREQUENTLY ASKED QUESTIONS		103
• **APPENDIX-4A**		109
▸ Self-Blood Glucose Monitoring Data (Diabetic Research)		111
▸ Self-Blood Glucose Monitoring Graphs (Diabetic Research)		122
▸ Recipes and Nutritional Composition of Meals Studied		128
▸ Chicken Meal, Tofu Meal, Fish Meal & Turkey Meal		129
○ REFERENCES		130

2nd Part of the Book Begins Here!
All About Food, Medication & Exercise To Fight & Control Diabetes!

	Page
	131
CHAPTER 5: HUMAN DIGESTIVE SYSTEM & KIDNEYS	133
▶ Introduction	135
▶ Human Digestive System (Description)	135
▶ Kidneys and the Urinary System (Description)	138
▶ Nutritional Breakdown of Foods	139
◯ REFERENCES	139
CHAPTER 6: HOW TO COUNT FOOD CALORIES?	141
▶ Concept of Calories	143
▶ READING LABELS & COUNTING CALORIES	143
▶ Example Calculation-I	143
How to Calculate Calories Offered by a Food Item	143
▶ Example Calculation-II	145
How to Calculate Calories of a Meal on Dinner Plate	145
▶ Distribution of Fat, Protein and Carbohydrate	146
▶ Nutritional Information of Liquid Egg Whites	147
▶ READING LABELS & COUNTING CALORIES (Continued)	149
▶ Using Calorie-Counting Tables	150
▶ Calculation of Protein, Fat and Carbohydrate	151
▶ Manipulation of Carbohydrate Content	152
▶ Accurate Carbohydrate Counting	153
▶ Is the Carbohydrate Correction Necessary?	153
▶ Is the Deduction of Fiber from Carbohydrate Necessary?	154
◯ REFERENCES	154
CHAPTER 7: FATS AND CHOLESTEROLS	155
▶ Fats, Saturated Fats, Unsaturated Fats	157
▶ Monounsaturated Fats, Polyunsaturated Fats	158
▶ Hydrogenated Fats	158
▶ Partially Hydrogenated Fats or Trans Fats	159
▶ What is Cholesterol?	160
▶ Normal Levels of Total Cholesterol, LDL, HDL	161
▶ CAUSES OF HIGH CHOLESTEROL IN PEOPLE WITH DIABETES	162
▶ HOW TO PREVENT HIGH CHOLESTEROL AND HEART DISEASE?	162
▶ Dr. Sweeny's Experiments on Diabetes	164
▶ Dr. T.J. Moore's Theory on Cholesterol	164
▶ Dr. Gabe Merkin's Report on Diabetes	165
◯ REFERENCES	165

	Page
CHAPTER 8: EAT WHOLE FOODS ONLY	167
Eat Whole Foods Only	169
Do Not Eat Processed Foods & Refined Foods	169
Examples of Whole Foods	169
Processed Foods	169
Examples of Processed Foods	170
Refined Foods	170
Examples of Refined Foods	170
Reasons Why You Have Fat in the Belly	171
Good Carbs Vs Bad Carbs	171
Nutrients are Needed for the Human Body Survival	172
Simple Carbohydrates Vs Complex Carbohydrates	173
List of Vegetables & Greens (Whole Foods) for Every Day Eating	173
REFERENCES	174
CHAPTER 9: DIABETES MEDICATIONS	175
Who Can Use Take Oral Medications & Who Can Use Insulin?	177
List of Oral Medications for Type 2 Diabetes	178
INSULIN THERAPY	179
Discovery of Artificial Insulin	179
Commercial or Synthetic Insulin	179
Types of Commercial or Symthetic Insulin	180
Handling and Storage of Insulin	181
Rotate Injection Sites, Or Face Lipohypertrophy!	181
Longer Needles, Or Shorter Needles?	181
Insulin Strength and Syringe Size	182
How to Prepare Insulin Injection (Illustrations)	184
How to Prepare Mixed Dose of Insulin Injection	185
Insulin Injection Sites	187
Self-Blood Glucose Tests and Finger Poking	188
INSULIN PUMPS (Medtronic, Tandem, OmniPod, Ypso Pump)	189
Insulin Inhalers, Patches and Capsules	192
Insulin Free World and Islet Transplantation	193
REFERENCES	194

	Page
CHAPTER 10: EXERCISE WITH DIABETES	195
▸ Introduction	197
▸ Advantages of Exercise	197
▸ How to Exercise?	198
▸ Energy Expenditure in Exercise (With Examples)	198
▸ Heart Rate (With Examples)	200
▸ Total Food Energy Requirement (With Example)	201
▸ How to Explain "3000 Calories = 1 Pound"?	201
▸ Operation of Treadmill	202
▸ Body Mass Index (BMI) With Sample Calculation	204
▸ Exercise and Sweating (Perspiration)	205
▸ Drink Purified Water Only (At Least 8 Cups A Day)	205
▸ PRECAUTIONS WHEN EXERCISING WITH DIABETES	206
▸ REFERENCES	206
CHAPTER 11: HEART DISEASE AND DIABETES	207
▸ Introduction	209
▸ CARDIOVASCULAR DISEASE	209
▸ FUNCTION OF THE HEART	210
▸ HEART VALVES AND VALVE DISEASE	211
▸ ATHEROSCLEROSIS AND ARTERIOSCLEROSIS	212
• An Illustration	212
▸ BLOOD PRESSURE (Explained)	213
▸ LOW BLOOD PRESSURE & HIGH BLOOD PRESSURE	213
▸ HEART ATTACK: SYMPTOMS AND TREATMENT	215
▸ STROKE: SYMPTOMS AND TREATMENT	215
▸ MEDICAL CHECK-UP AND DETECTION	216
▸ HEART DISEASE	217
• Angioplasty (Balloon, Stent and Laser)	217
• Angioplasty Procedure	218
• Bypass Surgery (Single, Double, Triple, Quadruple)	220
▸ DO DIABETICS HAVE TO GO THROUGH ALL THE ABOVE?	224
▸ THE AUTHOR SPEAKS OUT!	224
▸ NOTICE TO READERS & DISCLAIMER	226
▸ REFERENCES	226
CHAPTER 12: DIABETES GLOSSARY	227
▸ About the Author	231

Please visit www.mydiabetescontrol.com, and click on "Table of Contents".

About the Author

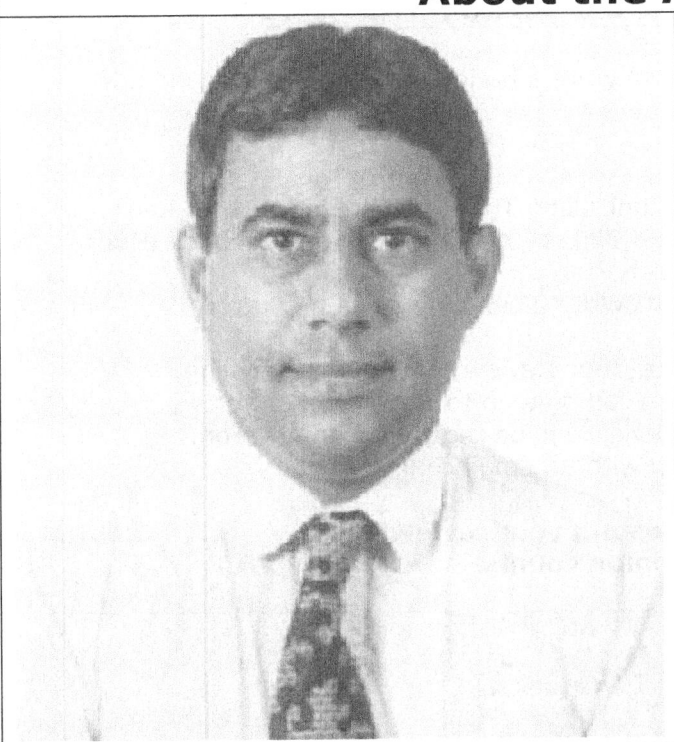

Rao Konduru, PhD (also called Dr. RK) published a book in the past titled "Permanent Diabetes Control", which earned immense respect and appreciation. Many people said it was a wonderful book. After suffering from a sudden heart attack, even though his left artery was 75% clogged and he could not walk a block due to severe angina pain, Dr. RK said "NO" to bypass surgery. He did what none of us would even think of doing. He simply relied on his natural self-prevention diet and exercise, and with it "reversed his critical diabetic heart disease in a matter of months", and developed a method to accomplish Permanent Diabetes Control. He proved to the medical community that a bypass surgery is unnecessary in most cases. He also came up with a trial and error procedure to determine the optimal insulin dose that would tightly control diabetes in 90 days, and would allow a diabetic person to live like a normal person for the rest of his/her life.

Please visit www.mydiabetescontrol.com, and read through the testimonials. Click on "Diabetic Research" button to see the Official Blood Test Results of Dr. RK. Notice the fact that he maintained his hemoglobin A1c level under 6.0% consistently. His personal best hemoglobin A1c level of 5.0% is an extraordinary result any diabetic person would hope to accomplish in a lifetime. Perhaps he is the only diabetic person living in this world now with "Permanent Diabetes Control".

Once again, quite recently health demons, such as uncontrollable weight gain, sleep apnea and chronic insomnia, came his way. Dr. RK did not give up, but persisted on discovering new, natural and effortless treatments of his own in reversing these most difficult disorders, through extensive reading, research, commitment, self-discipline and the strong desire to succeed. His extensive scientific research experience and his powerful knowledge helped him battle and combat these life challenges. He figured out their root causes, and developed natural yet powerful techniques to cure these health disorders. After losing 40 pounds of weight and 12 inches around the waist, Dr. RK successfully reversed his obesity, obstructive sleep apnea and chronic insomnia. He has carefully outlined and illustrated the methods he developed in three excellent books "Reversing Obesity, Reversing Sleep Apnea and Reversing Insomnia", so that others can benefit and be inspired to achieve similar results. His most recent book "Drinking Water Guide" is a 522-page wealth of information on drinking water for the rest of us.

- Prime Publishing Co.
www.mydiabetescontrol.com
www.reversinginsomnia.com
www.reversingsleepapnea.com
www.reversingsleepapnea.com/ebook2.html   (Reversing Obesity Book)
www.drinkingwaterguide.com   (The Most Important Book)

PLEASE WRITE A REVIEW ABOUT THIS BOOK

Now that you have read this book, please write a review about this book, and post your review on Amazon.

a. Please log into your Amazon account,
b. Search for this book "The Secret to Controlling Type 2 Diabetes (Author: Rao Konduru, PhD)", or by using ISBN # 9780973112054, and click on the book cover & scroll down,
c. Click on "Customer Reviews", click on "Write a customer review" button, and "Create Review" box pops up.
d. Kindly write your REVIEW in the Write-Your-Review box, type a Headline, and click on 5 stars overall rating (you can give up to 5 stars).
e. Click on "Submit" button, and your review will be registered on Amazon.
f. Amazon will acknowledge your review with an email confirmation!

Thanks for posting your review!
Your opinion counts!

YOUR OPINION COUNTS!

Kindle eBook Is Available on Amazon

You can read this book on your computer, laptop, tablet, e-reader, iPhone, or any Kindle device by purchasing Kindle eBook. It is available on Amazon. Please log into your Amazon account, and search for "The Secret to Controlling Type 2 Diabetes, Kindle eBook" or by using ASIN # B07RKJJHD2.

The End Of The Book "The Secret to Controlling Type 2 Diabetes"!

BEST WISHES!

Made in the USA
Middletown, DE
15 September 2020